THE
Egoscue Method
of Health
Through Motion

THE
Egoscue Method of Health of Health Through Motion

A Revolutionary Program
That Lets You Rediscover the Body's Power to
Protect and Rejuvenate Itself

Pete Egoscue
WITH
Roger Gittines

HarperCollins*Publishers*

FIRST EDITION

Illustrations by Hogie McMurtrie

Designed by Irving Perkins Associates

LIBRARY OF CONGRESS CATALOG CARD NUMBER 92-52558

ISBN 0-06-016881-1

92 93 94 95 96 AC/RRD 10 9 8 7 6 5 4 3 2 1

*This book is dedicated
to all those people who knew what was wrong with them,
but were told they did not;*

*to all those people who knew what to do about it,
but were told they could not;*

*and to all those people who tried to tell someone,
but were told they should not.*

Contents

List of Illustrations

CHAPTER SEVEN

Acknowledgments

It is every author's responsibility, and privilege, to publicly pay off outstanding IOUs before the curtain goes up on the main attraction. My biggest debt, which can never be fully repaid, is to the human body. The marvelous ingenuity and integrity of those 90-degree angles and parallel lines were there all along waiting to be recognized for what they really are—the motion-driven design of a healthy, functional man, woman, or child.

I am grateful to Harland for convincing me to give up the "milk run," to Diana for the delightful way she coaxes out excellence, and to the T.H.E. (Therapy, Health, Education) Clinic staff for proving every day to countless patients that the human spirit is what counts.

I worked closely with Roger Gittines on this book and made a friend; together we would like to thank our editor, Larry Ashmead, and his former assistant, Keonaona Peterson, who gave the manuscript thorough and professional treatment. The guidance and support of Susan Moldow of HarperCollins was also absolutely crucial. As always, our literary agent, Margret McBride, was there when it counted. There are many others, too many to name one by one. They read the manuscript in draft form, commented, critiqued, and acted as sounding boards. You know who you are, and know what good work you did. Thanks.

Foreword

by
Jack Nicklaus

In mid-1988 I was told by several doctors that unless I had either a discectomy or a discectomy plus a fusion, I probably would never play golf successfully again. I obviously did not want to accept the decision of surgery until I had exhausted all possible avenues of recovery. It was then that I ran into Pete Egoscue, and this foreword is to tell you how he has totally changed my life.

In chapter one of *Golf My Way,* I wrote, "I am not a believer in 'methods.' I'm a believer in fundamentals." That's still my view when it comes to golf, but as for an aching back and the rest of the body, I do believe in a method: the Egoscue Method. I have been to many specialists around the world, and yes, a few enabled me to achieve some marginal and temporary relief from pain. But never had I experienced such complete relief as I have by following the Egoscue Method. The fundamentals are sound, and it has worked for me since late 1988 when I put myself in Pete's hands after enduring several years of increasing amounts of pain, discomfort, and restricted movement caused by deteriorated disks in my lower back.

I was hurting. Take it from me, a sore back was a deterrent to my golf game, not to mention a good night's sleep. My ability to compete successfully, not only physically but mentally, was being undermined. From our first meeting, Pete's ideas and techniques made a difference, not that there was a quick fix. He warned me from the start that it would be some time before the good days outnumbered the bad. Even so, I was pleased to have the occasional good day—that was progress, in and of itself.

Pete told me the good days would become steadily more frequent, and indeed, that's what happened. As the pain decreased, I was able to start practicing again. Golf became fun again; I wasn't just going through the motions. On the average, I spend an hour and a half a day doing the exercises Pete recommended, and I have not missed a day since November of 1988. Sure enough, about seven or eight months after the workouts began, not only was I able to function, but my back stopped hurting also. You'll find the same exercises I used and more in the chapters ahead.

Pete gets results, without pills, manipulation, or a surgeon's scalpel. There are no gimmicks or shortcuts here; it just takes hard work and dedication. Unfortunately, many golfers seem to think that back pain or physical problems are inherent to the game, and they've gotten the idea that if they play through the pain, it will eventually go away. In fact, it seems that most athletes, whatever their sport, think that getting hurt and playing with pain are facts of life. I know that is not true from working with Pete and seeing the results he has achieved, not only with me but with many others as well.

I feel better than I have in years. It's not just the absence of pain, either. Pete has convinced me that many of the things we pass off as "age" or "an off day" are symptoms of the body slowly grinding to a halt through lack of motion. The Egoscue Method "jump starts" the body again, and that's why it feels good even if you've never had a back spasm in your life.

Pete has developed some extremely important concepts, all of them grounded on his uncanny talent for close observation and anatomical diagnosis. When Pete looks at the human body, his vision seems to go well beyond 20/20. I'm delighted that he has written this book. With the help of the Egoscue Method, we can all look forward to feeling better and performing better at whatever we do.

Introduction

What kind of a book is this? Fitness, alternative health care, diet, workout, back pain?

None of the above.

Those are all well-established genres, bristling with millions of words; as a part-time author and a full-time anatomical functionalist, I'm not interested in adding another sixty or seventy thousand to the total output.

This book is about responsibility. It's about you, and about the answer to a question I hear almost every day in my clinic: "How did I get in this condition?"

It's been asked so often over the years that I have to admit I don't remember the first time, but I do have a clear recollection of a woman from the Midwest, a lawyer, a wife, and a mother of two children, who was suffering from back spasms that prevented her from bending over and putting on her own shoes. "I wasn't born this way," she said, bewildered. "I haven't done anything stupid like go over Niagara Falls in a barrel. I'm just a normal person, doing normal things and it doesn't make any sense."

Three hours later I watched her lace her Reeboks. She looked up and there were tears in her eyes. "Thank you," she said.

"Thank yourself," I replied. "You made the pain go away. You took responsibility for your own health—not me."

And that message is the very heart and soul of this book. I want it understood up front because the idea makes or breaks what's come to be called the Egoscue Method, a system of diagnosis and treatment that has evolved out of my twenty-year study of human anatomy and anatomical function.

She got herself into that condition and she got herself out of it. So can you.

*   *   *

"I'm just a normal person, doing normal things . . ." comes awfully close to explaining—albeit enigmatically explaining—why it is that more than 35 million Americans suffer some form of back or joint pain. It also helps explain a lot of other things relating to our health, fitness, athletic skills, productivity on the job, performance in school, and happiness at home.

What's considered "normal" in the United States, Europe, Japan, and the rest of the industrialized world these days is really abnormal. For the first time in human history, most of us are living in an environment that does not require motion and movement for survival. We move very little compared to our ancestors. Yet the design of our "normal" bodies remains unchanged. And that design, both in terms of function and its continued maintenance, depends on motion.

In the pages ahead I will share with you my observations about the effects of this motionless world of ours. You'll soon start seeing and feeling those effects yourself. But I better quickly add that I'm not saying that by page two hundred you'll have sore knees and an aching shoulder. On the contrary. My objective is to provide my readers with the information and the expertise to allow them to make an educated judgment about what is happening to their own bodies. Then they can do what needs to be done, either to prevent the occurrence of back or joint pain and to improve overall fitness or to relieve symptomatic pain and restore lost functions.

And here I am back at the concept of responsibility. We are denying responsibility whenever that twinge in the knee is ignored, or when it sends us to the bathroom medicine cabinet for two aspirin tablets. Responsibility is denied when we blame the aching shoulder on tennis or "old age." All too often quick, costly cures and joint replacement surgery are used as ways to transfer responsibility. We must learn to recognize that the pain we feel, the stiffness, the lack of energy, the poor balance, the erratic concentration, or the inability to hit the long ball or the short putt aren't caused by the passing years, a second-rate golf club, or a bad day at the office: These are symptoms of dysfunctions brought on by lack of motion.

Taking responsibility means taking action. The Egoscue Method is a plan of action. There's no surgery, no drugs. You'll be able to recognize an everted foot or elevated hip for what it really is—a symptom of *correctable* dysfunction.

I'll show you how to "turn back the clock" on your body. One of my patients, a champion athlete, recently called to say how thrilled he was that his right shoulder was hurting. He said he could feel a burning sensation.

"What's so thrilling about that?" I asked.

"My shoulder hasn't done that since I was sixteen years old," he said.

He was in touch with a body that had been lost since the days when he was beginning to rewrite the record books and being hailed as a boy wonder.

There will be a series of exercises that will allow you to do the same thing.

But—the Egoscue Method simply won't work if you believe that someone or something else is responsible for your health. The buck cannot be handed off to me, or to a physician, a chiropractor, a drug company, or a pair of fancy running shoes.

Until you recognize the need, the absolute requirement for taking responsibility, you will not succeed. Once you do accept the responsibility, however, the Egoscue Method never fails. Never. No drugs, no surgery, no machines, no miracles. Just You. A normal person, doing normal things.

A sweeping claim, but I can make it in confidence because I see what happens every day in my clinic in San Diego. Hardly a week goes by without telephone calls or personal visits from physicians, chiropractors, or physical therapists who have heard about the Egoscue Method and want to see it firsthand. I welcome them all because my objective is to revolutionize diagnostic and therapeutic technique worldwide. And even better, I want to make those revolutionary techniques largely irrelevant because the Egoscue Method has proven itself again and again as a powerful and effective preventive strategy.

Pain and dysfunction are not inevitable.

The method is derived from more than two decades of research and rigorous therapeutic application that began when I was wounded while serving as a Marine infantry officer in Vietnam in 1969.

For a time I was immobilized in a military hospital, and it struck me just how quickly one loses physical functions under those circumstances. There seemed to be almost a direct correlation between lack of motion and lack of function, yet conventional wisdom decreed that it's best to rest an injured joint, muscle, or limb. At what point, I wondered, did the convalescence contribute to the dysfunction?

The intensive recovery and rehabilitation process that followed introduced me to a professional discipline that I chose to follow as a career when I left the Marines after eleven years of service. Ever since, I have been totally immersed in biomechanics and functional anatomy.

What I've learned would probably fill the pages of ten books, and perhaps someday I'll get around to writing them. But the most important lesson of all is the central premise of this book: We can't live without adequate motion, and our motionless lifestyle is nothing less than a slow death.

The signs of dysfunction are all around us. Look. The man standing at the corner waiting for the traffic light to change is rubbing the backs of his hands. Perhaps he's nervous. But there's another possibility: Perhaps he's reacting to the symptoms of a rounded shoulder, which in a month or two will be diagnosed as carpal tunnel syndrome. Notice, I said a symptom. Carpal tunnel syndrome is a symptom of a shoulder dysfunction, not a wrist, forearm, or elbow problem.

My mother suffered from migraine headaches, and those were also symptomatic. Today in the grocery store near my clinic I see people pushing their shopping carts whose heads hang down and forward like hers did. I watched my mother's health deteriorate as she and her doctors treated symptoms, not the underlying problems. Tortured by her migraines, she would spend days in bed with the window shades drawn. I sensed that she was slowly slipping toward death, but there was nothing I could do about it. I'd beg her to get out of bed. One day, in exasperation with me she said, "You just don't understand . . . maybe someday you will."

It's too late for my mother. But I can say this: I understand. I've made it my life's work to understand.

Join me, and in this book I'll introduce you to techniques that can easily restore lost functions by reintroducing the right kinds and the right amount of movement.

If you're not in pain, so much the better. I'll guide you through the steps to increasing your energy levels, maximizing your physical and mental capabilities, and protecting yourself against accidents and future dysfunction.

Along the way I will mix in some evolutionary concepts, cultural history, and social patterns. We'll talk sports and leisure, discuss children and the elderly, examine the "motionless" workplace and home.

In the end, I hope that you too will understand.

THE
Egoscue Method of Health Through Motion

A DIFFERENT DISCLAIMER

Ours is a highly litigious society. Which means, in plain English, we like to sue each other, blame each other, transfer responsibility to others.

Since, as you'll see, responsibility is a continuing theme of this book, the space which is usually reserved for what the lawyers refer to as the "disclaimer" is being used to make an additional and, I believe, more important point.

You've seen the words many times: "The following material is not intended as a substitute for the advice of a physician. The reader should consult a physician before embarking on this or any health program . . ."—or words to that effect. The all-purpose liability firebreak.

Disclaimers are a legal necessity, but they are a cop-out. This material is no substitute for the reader taking responsibility for his or her own health. Therefore, I have an important recommendation to make: If you really need a disclaimer, close the book and put it back on the shelf unread.

I hope you don't—because what I have to say in the pages ahead will change your life.

—PETE EGOSCUE

1

For Form's Sake

Imagine a man and a woman. Imagine a child, and a family with its concentric rings of youthful dreams and mature wisdom.

Does a picture come to mind? I'll bet one does, and I'd say it's probably a *motion* picture.

The man, the woman, and the child, all the generations reaching back at least ten thousand years, are in motion. Walking on a beach; running down a winding road at sunset; climbing a staircase under a crystal chandelier.

From birth to death, we never stop moving. Even asleep, we toss and turn; the heart beats. Motion—that's what the human body is all about.

If you thumbed through these pages the way I always do before I buy a book, you might have come to the conclusion that you're going to be reading about how to cure back, knee, or shoulder pain; how to play better golf, run faster, work more productively, or take a few inches off your hips.

All that's in here. But between the lines, above and behind the lines, is a premise that is so important, so basic, that I can't afford to treat it with subtlety. Just as I do with the patients who come to my clinic, I'm going to lay it on the line: *You are not moving enough to keep your body and overall health from deteriorating.* And when you do move, because this "motion starvation" is acute, the movement violates the design of the body with every step you take.

How do I know this without ever setting eyes on you? I'm taking an educated guess; one that's educated by about twenty-

1

two years of experience as an anatomical functionalist. I've treated thousands of people who the demographers would identify as fitting the profile of those most likely to read this book: the educated and middle-aged, professional and recreational athletes, parents and teachers, white collar professionals and medical specialists, the elderly, and a huge number of individuals from every walk of life who suffer some form of joint or muscular pain.

I have learned that out of all those people, only a tiny fraction move enough to beat the overwhelming odds that one day this motionless modern lifestyle will catch up with them.

Here's another thing that I've learned: There's a lot written about dwindling nonrenewable, essential resources, and for man, motion is just that—an absolutely essential resource. It makes us strong, active, intelligent, and healthy. It renews and is renewable. But motion, as a resource, is becoming scarcer all the time. The way we live in the last decade of the twentieth century in the United States, Western Europe, Japan, and other parts of the industrialized world does not supply or require sufficient movement to maintain the body's health and well-being.

We know that the body needs minimum daily requirements of vitamins, minerals, protein, and water. There are other necessities determined by biological fiat as well: shelter, warmth, space, companionship. If there is a "she who must be obeyed" (Rumpole fans take note), *she* is biology.

Disobedience to the biological imperatives results in disaster and death.

Have you ever stopped to think that movement is as much of a biological imperative as food and water? It is. There was a time, and not long ago, when it was easy, instinctive, to obey the biological imperative of motion. Man moved because he had to. Not anymore. Survival doesn't depend on motion. We can sit at a desk, sit in a car, sit in front of the TV set, and live the "good life."

But we are paying for this "good" life of ours with illness, disability, pain, and despair. What all of us must do is deliberately and systematically get our bodies back in motion despite a modern lifestyle that discourages movement, and even encourages us to believe that we can survive and prosper as sedentary beings who treat motion as an inconvenience that can be minimized with the help of technology. Just as we would perish without food and water, we will perish once our bodies are deprived of the movement necessary to maintain our vital physiological systems.

As a species, particularly those of us who live in the industrialized world, we are getting closer and closer to the edge, and that's why I developed the Egoscue Method. It is a way to provide each person with sufficient motion, motion that is no longer built into the daily pattern of our lives the way it was just a few decades ago; and it is a way back to motion that is in accord with the body's design requirements. Motion doesn't just happen anymore. From now on we'll have to work at it. The Egoscue Method is your tool box.

STEP BY STEP

I mentioned design requirements. I'll explain what I mean. Most of us have disobeyed the biological imperative of movement for so long that when we do put our bodies in motion, what should be motion of the most routine sort causes pain or forces the body to compensate in ways that drain away our energy levels, undermine our physical and athletic ability, and will one day bring on pain. The design of the body is being violated with every step we take, and that simply does not have to happen.

THE REAL EXPERTS

I want to explain the Egoscue Method to you, so that you can live the method and make it work. But we can't just leap right in and start doing a series of exercises. There's more to the method than a workout program or a series of pain suppression procedures. First, we'll need some background on human anatomy and evolution to understand the body's design, functions, and requirements.

In my clinic, I've found that too many patients honestly believe that their musculoskeletal system is so complicated that a) it's fragile and prone to breakdown, and b) it can't be comprehended by laymen.

Let's start, as we do in the clinic, by unlearning a demoralizing lesson taught to us by the "experts." I hear this comment all the time, it could almost be the mantra of the twentieth century: "It can't be that simple." We don't believe our own eyes and instincts anymore. Motion? It can't be that simple.

I suppose the preoccupation with complexity is a by-product of education and knowledge. The more we know, the more we must know. Technology adds to the confusion by accelerating the learning process and removing us from a direct, hands-on relationship with many facets of life that were once readily experienced and understood. The interest in natural childbirth and the hospice movement for the terminally ill are attempts at reclaiming birth and death from technology. But those are small toe-holds.

Technology has many long, powerful tentacles reaching out to grasp the great and small aspects of life. I think it's a shame, and more than a little disturbing, that in a few more years cars will be so technologically advanced that it will be impossible for drivers to repair their own vehicles. Another fragment of self-sufficiency will disappear and at that point transportation will become a mystery, complicated and incomprehensible to all but a few.

I can just imagine the typical driver of the year 2020: "Why doesn't the car start?"

"Maybe it's out of gas."

"It can't be that simple."

It's an ironic twist. We've become smart enough to realize we aren't smart enough. We've been outsmarted by the experts and by the technology they serve.

I am about to reclaim a small piece of captured territory from the experts and from technology. Small, but big enough for a kingdom. The human body.

Its royal motto is a variation on the old populist battle cry, "Every man a king." When it comes to the human body, *everyone* is an expert. We don't need technology to understand our own bodies and the biological imperatives that drive them. By tapping our own expertise, we can unlock the maximum potential that lies within each of us, with immediate and enormous benefit to the lives we lead, the work we accomplish, the sports we play.

THE BODY OF KNOWLEDGE

In all the years that I have been helping people overcome pain and physical dysfunction, and to make the most of their potential and talent, there has not been a single individual who could not tell me what was going on inside that marvelous machine we call the human body.

Most did not have a command of the specialized vocabulary familiar to the medical community, but they knew.

"After my wife and I had kids there was no time. None," a patient told me at our first meeting. "I stopped doing a lot of things. Softball, for one, went by the boards."

"Play a lot?" I asked.

"Before we got so busy it was a couple of times a week. I thought I'd go out for the company team this spring but after the first game I started with this stupid stiff neck. Guess I'm a little rusty."

Rusty. He knew, and so do you.

However, the lack of a specialized vocabulary and formal schooling makes us uneasy, living as we do in a complicated world; there's a tendency to defer to those who know all the right words and phrases, and have all the impressive letters after their names.

Right here, right now I want to share with you my experience. The design of the human body is so complete, so complex in its interrelationships, so prepared for its world of motion that it allows for its function to be very simple. Foolproof, really. And it's a good thing. We don't have the brain power to consciously oversee incredibly intricate processes like digestion and respiration and locomotion. All we have to do is move and keep on moving until we die. Along the way, poetry gets written and pyramids are built.

THE BONES: ANATOMY WITHOUT TEARS

The complexity of the body's design is fascinating, and that's precisely why we get so confused. There are 639 individual muscles (approximately 400 skeletal muscles) and over 200 bones in an adult human. A medium-sized muscle contains about 10 million muscle cells, which means a total of 6 billion in the overall musculature. These are described in the anatomy textbooks as contractile cells, because they are composed of bundles of parallel fibrils—some thick (myosin), some thin (actin)—which interact chemically and mechanically. Energized by calcium ions, the myosin fibrils rake or pull their actin counterparts upward to produce a visible shortening of the muscle tissue.

The fibrils under magnification appear to contain a series of ten light and dark "boxes." The transfer of fluid among the boxes with resultant swelling and relaxation—sort of like the individual cylinders of an internal combustion engine firing in sequence—is what drives the muscle cell. Add this all up and we have a body which is propelled by a 24-trillion cylinder engine. Now there's horsepower!

In just one paragraph, I went from 639 muscles—a daunting study in their own right—to 24 trillion "cylinders." What would happen if I began to focus in on each of the cylinders? I would be drawn ever deeper into a labyrinth of incredible complexity, which is precisely what has happened to medical science. Lost in the maze is the simple imperative of the body's function: movement. Once we are disoriented and demoralized by all the twists and turns and blind alleys, movement seems inconsequential and hardly worth bothering about.

What a mistake. We get obsessed with the form, layers and layers of form, and forget about the function; forget that function dictates form. In other words, movement is a determining factor in how we look and how we feel. When we set out to discover what's wrong or right with the body, isn't that the logical place to begin?

I'll show you what I mean. But I'm not going to do it with a traditional skeletal chart, which is like trying to learn how to type by studying the schematics of a typewriter. I prefer to use a simple stick figure instead; it doesn't confuse with detail but shows overall design. You can draw it yourself on a scrap of paper: a small circle for the head—go ahead—put a smile on it and a couple of eyes; beneath the head, by about a half inch or so, add two points on the same horizontal line to form the left and right shoulders; a bit farther down the sheet put two more points in, the right and left hips exactly under the shoulders; beneath those, draw two points for the right and left knees; and finish with a final set of points for the right and left ankles and feet, again right under the knees.

As drawn, the perspective is head on, eyeball to eyeball. Not at all complicated, is it? If you draw straight lines through the horizontals and verticals, a series of right angles emerges, as shown in figure 1. Those right angles are the key to understanding the body's design.

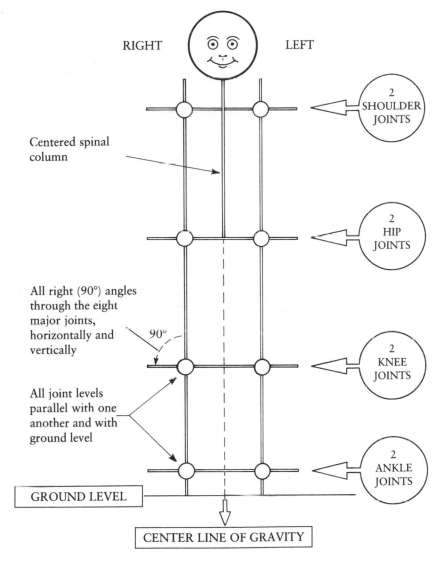

RIGHT · · LEFT

2 SHOULDER JOINTS

Centered spinal column

2 HIP JOINTS

All right (90°) angles through the eight major joints, horizontally and vertically   90°

2 KNEE JOINTS

All joint levels parallel with one another and with ground level

2 ANKLE JOINTS

GROUND LEVEL

CENTER LINE OF GRAVITY

Figure 1
FRONT VIEW: THE FUNCTIONAL DESIGN POSTURE

The joints at the shoulders, hips, knees, and ankles maintain their right angles no matter what position the body assumes (short of a violent, wrenching contortion that destroys this natural design). The right angles give the body great strength and durability. We stand upright in the presence of gravity carrying our own weight on two feet—an achievement we take for granted, yet one unique to our species. What's more, we are capable not only of defying gravity but of moving at the same time, and that with speed, agility, and endurance. From an architectural standpoint it is the equivalent of constructing a thirty-story office tower that could compete in the Boston Marathon.

We may not all have "the right stuff," but we all do have the right angles, or at least our anatomical design calls for them. Those right angles provide a most important piece of anatomical information about the body and its functions: We are upright, load bearing, all-terrain, all-weather *motion* machines.

If man ever goes the way of the dinosaurs and our planet is visited by extraterrestrial paleontologists searching for clues as to the identity of Earth's former inhabitants, they would surely recognize (just as we recognized from the shape and size of the fossil remains that pterodactyls were designed to fly) that whatever else the mysterious bipeds may have been capable of doing—speaking, tool making, reasoning—they were intended to walk, to run, to jump, to dance—to move.

What I call "the four socket position," the right angles at the shoulders, hips, knees, and ankles, is irrefutable evidence that man was designed to move.

Move we do, and move we must.

ON TWO FEET

The extraterrestrial paleontologists would probably also be fascinated by man's spinal column. It is an engineering marvel. Figure 2 is a side view of the stick figure, which stops being a stick figure when the spine is considered. Our "backbone" forms a gentle S-curve which distributes the weight evenly from head to hip. The movement of the individual vertebra allows for four degrees of movement, front to back. This movement along the S-curve effectuates weight distribution: It's a balancing act. Eight or nine degrees of movement would make us top heavy; the head would roll forward and we would fold over. Conversely, with only two or three degrees of movement we would be stiff and unbalanced, and better off closer to the ground where our lower torso could compensate for the immobility of the upper body.

FORM AND FUNCTION: BONE AND MUSCLE

The spine is such a work of art, it's tempting to conclude that anything so complicated has got to be subject to Murphy's Law: What can go wrong will go wrong. But that's not the case; if the

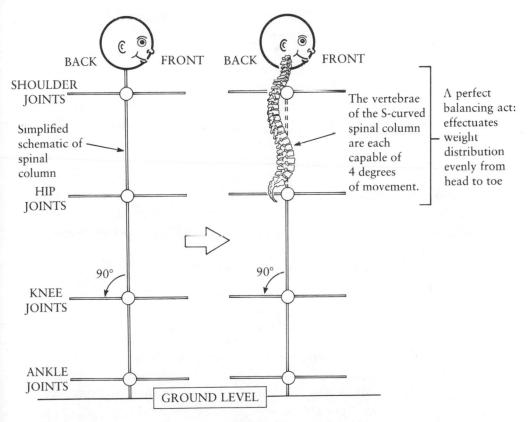

Figure 2
SIDE VIEW: THE FUNCTIONAL DESIGN POSTURE

spine had been prone to breakdown, the human species would never have made it this far.

Here again the spine's complex form supports a simple function. The spine and all the body's joints are there to participate in a range of motion—design motion—that is easy to catalog. We can bend at the waist, twist and turn to the right and left, raise our knees upward toward the chest, and so on. Each design motion, in addition, comes naturally. It's not taught like learning to walk a tightrope or play the violin. The environment demands a given response from the body, and at first haltingly, then with growing strength and assurance, we walk and run and jump. The more we do it, the stronger, more agile, and faster we become. And the reverse is also true: The less we do, the weaker, less agile, and slower we become.

We are built to walk and run and jump because we are the descendants of primitive hunter-gatherers. Those are survival skills. The body's form is determined by its functions. In other words, who we are is decided by what we must do to continue to exist: Form follows function.

There's another old saying, "Necessity is the mother of invention." Well, the human body was invented by necessity. Primitive man either moved or perished. The design of the body was "invented" to satisfy that requirement. Today, the design is unaltered, but what has changed is necessity. Technology has intervened; we are not moving a body that was intended for movement, and which depends on that movement for its continued operation and maintenance. The body knows this and tells us the facts of life.

How? The most dramatic way is with pain.

A BILATERAL MACHINE

To understand the source of the pain, let's leave the hunter-gatherers and return to the stick figure. Figure 3 shows us that the four socket position, the right angles, comes in matched sets. We have four on the right side of the body and four on the left. As a matter of fact, we have two of everything. A right hand, a left hand; right wrist, left wrist; right elbow, left elbow. It's as if we are Siamese twins sharing the same head, vertebrae, and internal organs. The body has bilateral function. For want of a better word, let's just say it's bifunctional: The right and left sides are designed to do the same things, and the component parts—bones, muscles, ligaments, tendons—are identical. Not vaguely similar, *identical.*

Nearly every day I have someone come into my clinic and, in so many words, inform me that they are the exception to this rule of bifunctionality. "My right arm is longer than my left arm," they say. Or, "I've always had to get my new slacks altered because one leg is shorter than the other." I have heard it enough times that I could reply in my sleep.

"Oh, really? Did you suffer a traumatic injury to the growth plate as a child before you attained your full adult height?"

"Well, no . . . I don't think so."

"Hmmm, childhood injuries—and I mean big-time hurt, not minor bumps and jolts—are the primary cause of an asymmetrical skeletal structure. And one person out of several million may be affected by a birth defect, a statistically minuscule number." I usually get a blank look at that point, and I go on to suggest the possibility that it isn't that one leg is shorter than the other, but rather something that is happening to one hip which isn't happening to the other.

Notice that I didn't say that one hip is *different.* It isn't. The architecture of the body is designed to be bifunctional. In their form, both hips are alike because they were intended to perform exactly the same function, that is, to bear weight in an upright position and to move.

THE BODY AS A UNIT

There is one more concept that needs to be examined in order to gain a working knowledge of human anatomy as it pertains to the Egoscue Method and to you and your body. It relates directly to bifunctionality. If one side of the body is just like the other side, and since the two halves form a whole, it is logical to assume that we are designed to function as a unit.

Our old friend Mr. Bones, who makes a cameo appearance in every basic anatomy text, is the best example. He is a single unit from head to foot, as is obvious in the words of the song, "the hip bone is connected to the thigh bone. . . ."

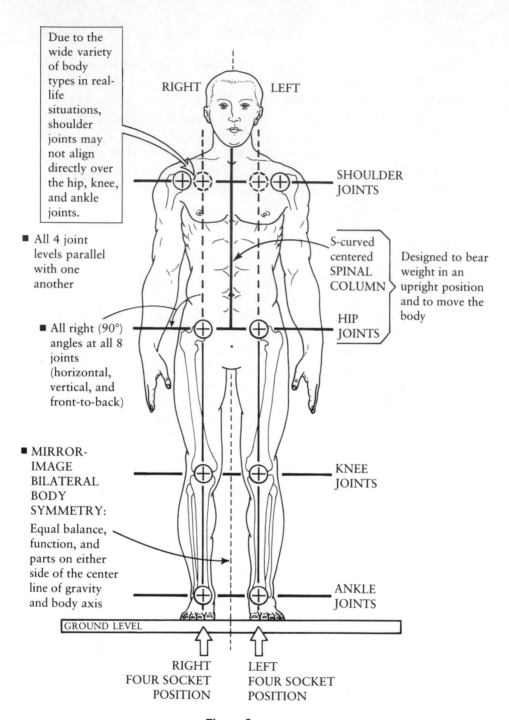

Due to the wide variety of body types in real-life situations, shoulder joints may not align directly over the hip, knee, and ankle joints.

RIGHT   LEFT

SHOULDER JOINTS

■ All 4 joint levels parallel with one another

S-curved centered SPINAL COLUMN

Designed to bear weight in an upright position and to move the body

HIP JOINTS

■ All right (90°) angles at all 8 joints (horizontal, vertical, and front-to-back)

■ MIRROR-IMAGE BILATERAL BODY SYMMETRY:

Equal balance, function, and parts on either side of the center line of gravity and body axis

KNEE JOINTS

ANKLE JOINTS

GROUND LEVEL

RIGHT FOUR SOCKET POSITION

LEFT FOUR SOCKET POSITION

Figure 3

Why stop at the thigh? Proceed a bit farther down the leg to the knee, and we encounter the original synchronizing gear. It sits there between the hip and the foot. The knee design is too complex to duplicate—even though we try—but like the rest of the body, it is functionally very simple. This gear keeps us from walking like the Tin Man in the *Wizard of Oz*. The knee does what the hip and the foot tell it to do. Therefore hip, knee, and foot are a unit. This unit, or whole, is the sum of its parts. Impairment of one affects them all—not to mention *repairment*. A unit is a unit and must be treated like one. In time, many patients who have had hip replacement surgery start experiencing knee problems. Separatism may work in the former Soviet Union or Eastern Europe, but not when it comes to our musculoskeletal units.

THE ONE AND ONLY DESIGN

Anatomically, the body is very democratic: All men and women are created equal. We have the same basic design, the same bones, the same muscles, the same nerves. What we do with what we've got makes the difference. The weight lifter's huge muscle mass is primarily the result of his exercise regimen, and he would relatively quickly become a ninety-pound weakling if he stopped moving.

A few years ago, I told a group of young women who were training to run in the New York Marathon about this anatomical equality and they didn't want to believe it.

"We've been hearing since we were little girls," one of them said, "that we're built differently."

"Think of it this way," I replied, "if form follows function what is the one function that men and women do not share?" It took less than a nanosecond to get an answer.

"Childbearing."

"Right. The female anatomical form primarily differs from the male in the pelvis and the hips. A woman's pelvis is slightly wider than a man's, but this alone has no functional consequences. The big difference is where the femur bone fits into the socket of the hip joint. It goes in at a reduced angle compared to a man's. The difference in angle allows a woman's pelvis to flare into the birthing position and return to normal once the child is delivered." I stopped and pointed at the one member of the group who was the most dedicated runner. "Is that going to impact on Jill's time? Not unless she's planning to have a kid right there on the finish line."

MUSCLE MECHANICS

In figure 4 we're really looking at a map, and you can trace the muscular and skeletal roads that link the shoulders with the feet.

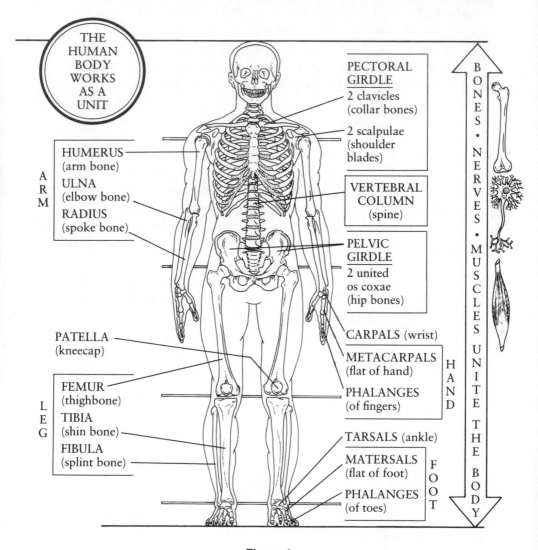

Figure 4

Those bones, nerves, and muscles form a highway system that unites the body. There are no dead ends; each of the routes interconnects.

These muscles and nerves add another dimension to the body's unitary design. Indeed, without them, and without tendons and ligaments, the unit would fall apart. There is, however, a leader of the pack. The muscles run the show. The bones do what the muscles and nerves tell them to do.

By definition a skeletal muscle is a tissue composed of an assortment of different muscle cell types, long and cylindrical in shape, striated, and all capable of contracting when stimulated. We don't need to know much more than that. Actually, what most people think they know about their muscles is just plain wrong anyway.

Frequently, runners and other athletes will tell me "I stretch before I work out every day."

It may feel like it, but that's not what is actually happening. Muscles do not stretch in the way lycra outfits stretch. A skeletal muscle is attached to a bone at both ends and always stays attached. The overall design length remains roughly constant as it elongates and contracts. Muscles change length through a complex mechanical and chemical interaction between thin filaments and thick fibrils of a muscle fiber. Like a ratchet mechanism, the fibrils and filaments pull together and the muscle contracts. When a muscle elongates, or, as we commonly say "stretches," the ratchet is reversed and the fibrils and filaments slowly let go of each other. This elongation of the muscle allows it to return to its design length.

If you bend at the waist to touch your toes and your hamstrings and glutes are "stiff," it is not that the muscles are shorter than they were last week. Here's what's happening: What we regard as stretching is an important aspect of the body's fail-safe system that protects it from events that would restrict the ability to move. Stiffness or resistance when we walk or run or bend is similar to the message a ball player gets when he is chasing a fly ball and crosses the warning pad—Watch it! You're approaching the center field wall. In the same way, the muscles are telling us that they are approaching the limit of what they regard as normal motion, beyond which damage might be done.

To understand how it works, visualize the muscle as an organized collection of fibers with spindles and receptors strategically placed among them. The spindles and receptors are sensors relaying information to the central nervous system about the fiber's movement. If our movements regularly engage all of our muscle groups, then our body easily accommodates whatever physical demands we put on it, squatting, jumping, bending; all in a day's work.

Conversely, if our muscle's range of motion is restricted on a consistent basis, by sitting, driving, and loafing, the muscle adapts to this position. When the muscle is then asked to move, the spindles and receptors are caught by surprise. They simply do not know what to make of the activity being performed. Therefore, the musculoskeletal computer, to use another helpful metaphor, warns the body to be careful by generating resistance to movement.

In the most extreme cases, if the spindles and receptors panic because the motion of the muscle is too sudden or violent, they trigger what's known as the stretch reflex, which orders the muscle to contract to protect itself. The stretch reflex is akin to what happens when we accidentally touch a hot stove. We flinch. The muscles contract immediately, and sometimes with enough force to do damage.

We see many patients in my clinic with vacation-related injuries. People sit around for most of the year and then for a week or two expect to pick up where they left off running or hitting a tennis ball or sliding into home plate. But muscles adjust to inactivity very quickly. It's a way to conserve energy. If we're at a desk for eight hours the muscle concludes that it is there to stay. Stand up to go home and there's stiffness. Stop at the basketball court along the way and suddenly jump for a slam-dunk and there's pain. Again, it's a message that should not be ignored. The muscle is telling us that normal motion—and the spindles and receptors have concluded that normal means sitting at a desk—is being pushed beyond safe limits.

A key thing to remember is that the body continually monitors its motion and adjusts accordingly. The number-one priority is to keep the musculoskeletal system intact. When it senses danger, such as movement that could destroy a joint, there is an almost instantaneous assessment and the least damaging option is selected, that is, the muscle pulls or tears like a circuit breaker tripping before a power surge burns down the house. The problem is that our circuit breakers are being set off these days by demands—climbing a flight of stairs, bending down for the morning newspaper—that were once routine.

SOME NERVES

Muscular pain is nothing more, really, than a message. We have to learn how to decode it. The code is being sent to the brain via the individual filaments of the central nervous system. For the most part, this system is foolproof, which modern man finds hard to believe. Just as we must learn to accept that there is nothing wrong with the design of the skeletal system, it is necessary to reject the automatic assumption that if there is pain, and the bones and muscles seem okay, then there is a "problem" with the nervous system. Simple process of elimination, right?

Not necessarily. There is too much emphasis put on what are known as neurological impacts. I hear a lot about neuropathy from my new patients, basically an interruption of neural function—the message flow being cut off—by disease or injury. It happens, but not that often.

People come to me and say that they have been told that their constant pain and numbness in the feet and hands are caused by neuropathy. One woman was convinced that her cold feet were caused by neuropathy until I asked her to spend fifteen minutes doing a simple exercise.

"What about your feet?" I asked when she was done. She looked puzzled. "Are they still cold?"

"I don't think so," she replied tentatively, wiggling her toes.

"What about your neuropathy? That exercise worked on your hip. It didn't have anything to do with the nerves."

"Maybe the workout . . ." the patient stopped in midsentence. "It wasn't neuropathy," she said.

That was the last we heard about neuropathy, and the last of her cold feet as well. I think she was in awe of the terminology. Sounds bad, doesn't it? Neuropathy. Not nearly as impressive as being informed that your symptoms are caused by lack of motion, which has transformed the leg muscles into Silly Putty and, in turn, signaled the nervous system that it is no longer necessary to enervate muscles or pump much oxygenated blood into the lower extremities since the flaccid muscles aren't in need of the oxygen. The cold or numbness is a signal—the nerves are working just fine—that the muscle is shut down.

And that is one of the primary functions of the nervous system. It is supposed to act as an early warning system. The inactive muscle is in the first stages of dying. The nerves announce that fact to the brain, and it then tells you to do something about it. If you were standing in a snowbank in the middle of January, you would stomp your feet and jump up and down to get the blood flowing. Since the diagnosis is neuropathy, however, you just sit there with your cold feet.

When hard or soft tissue starts pushing against a nerve there is pain (or numbness, the absence of pain); a warning message. The phone is ringing, and if we say "never mind, it is neuropathy calling," we're going to miss an important call.

Physicians have learned to recognize some of the calls. When the sciatic nerve rings and there's pain shooting down the leg, they know one of the disks in the vertebrae is impinging on the nerve root.

If nerves, muscles, and bones add up to a single unit, the idea of going after one of the unit's components doesn't make much sense. Just as the sciatic nerve isn't causing the pain, neither is the disk. Yet the common surgical practice is to remove the disk and fuse the spine. The call got through, but the message was misunderstood. The disk may be gone, but the problem still remains elsewhere in the unit.

HALF AND HALF

I have to bear down on this concept of the body as a unit because too often it is forgotten or ignored by people who should know better. Right-handed tennis players come into my clinic and wonder why I have them work on the left side of the body (and vice versa for the lefties).

"It's my right shoulder that hurts," one red-hot teenage star informed me. "Let's not waste time on the left."

"You leave the left shoulder in the locker room when you play?" I asked.

He thought I was being a wise guy, and I was. The point, however, was this: He spent years, thousands of hours, developing just one side of his body. One wrist, one elbow, one shoulder, one hip, one knee, one ankle, and one foot. Half a body was doing all the work—lunging, hitting, stretching, balancing, pivoting. The other side was just there.

It wasn't the fault of tennis. It was his fault and the fault of the youngster's coaches. The body does its damndest to do what we tell it to do. When the pectoralis major, the anterior portion of the deltoid and the biceps brachii, can't handle the forehand stroke of the tennis racquet the way they're supposed to, the body will enlist other muscles to help out. After a while the body starts looking like a lifeboat with all the passengers crowded onto one side. The boat rolls over; the body starts hurting.

My mutant teenage tennis whiz was so talented he might have gotten away with playing that way. But he had to leave the court every now and then to eat and sleep and do other normal things. Every time he walked up a set of stairs he was in agony because the muscles on his right side were telling him in no uncertain terms that they were sick and tired of doing all the work, and the muscles on the left side were seconding the motion by announcing that they didn't do stair climbing.

There's a happy ending to this story because the young man opted not to have surgery on his shoulder—the problem wasn't in his shoulder—and instead to reengage his left side. He's out on the circuit playing competitive tennis today. When I think of his experience I have to ask, is it any wonder that dozens of marvelous young tennis players are hurting and headed for retirement before they're twenty?

The answer to that question springs out of an image created by the late Italo Calvino, the Italian short story writer. Calvino wrote a novella titled *The Cloven Viscount*. It was about an Italian nobleman who returned from the Napoleonic wars after being split in half by a cannonball. His two halves operated separately, doing good and evil. A great story; a great image.

What's not so great, though, is that we're creating a generation of young "cloven" athletes, talented men and women who have been trained and encouraged to throw away half their bodies. When the cheering stops, their reward is pain, numbing fatigue, lost potential, and early retirement.

IN THE PICTURE

For every "cloven" athlete there are thousands of people who share similar disabilities and never set foot on a tennis court or a football field. For them, the simplest acts of everyday life—standing up, sitting down, bending over, turning the head to the left or right—are unnatural acts.

The pain they feel is confirmation that an unnatural act is taking place. Pain is the body's way of getting our attention; from "Pssst!" to a thunder clap. And each one of these warnings comes with a picture so that we'll understand the meaning.

The body isn't taking any chances. At the same time a dysfunction manifests itself in the form of pain, it is also visible to the eye. But most of us refuse to look at the truth. We assume that things like everted feet, rounded shoulders, one leg being shorter than the other are nothing more than heredity or birth defects. However, all of these characteristics are *symptoms*.

Take for example the "short" leg of the patient whose visit to my clinic I described earlier in this chapter. If we had measured both legs from the heel up to the ball of the femur, which fits into the hip joint's socket, the length would have been the same for each. Yet one leg definitely looked longer. The discrepancy was caused by the man bearing most of his weight on the left or "longer" leg, which, in the course of doing the extra work, has shifted the pelvis vertically and horizontally. One side of the pelvis, the ilium, has been pulled downward, and the other one pushed upward (and forward).

But isn't this a distinction without a difference? Whatever the cause, the effect is a "short" leg.

I'll answer one rhetorical question with another: Why should we live with half a body when we don't have to? In a mature adult there's no way medical science can make a truly short leg grow to its proper length. The treatments are palliatives. But the unnatural acts that deprived the man of the use of his gait muscles can be easily eliminated by reintroducing his body to proper movement, to natural acts.

PAST PERFECT

Like the young tennis player's aching right shoulder and the man with the "short" leg, the body's messages and the accompanying pictures are widely misunderstood. Sore knees do not mean that jogging is bad for the body; low back pain is not caused by too much golf. There is a growing list of activities and situations that we are too fragile to participate in, or so it seems from the warning signs that are being posted on various sports, fitness routines, pieces of office equipment, and occupations.

I don't accept that today's men and women, descendants of hunter-gatherers, people who just a few thousand years ago walked and ran for miles each day in sun and rain, heat and cold, over rocks and through the brush, are too frail to enjoy an evening jog in the park or to operate the keyboard of a computer.

From an evolutionary standpoint, a thousand years—make it five thousand—amounts to about a day and a half, if that. And if we have permanently lost our ability to walk and run and endure without pain in such a short time span, either our understanding of the principles of evolution is totally cockeyed or we are headed for extinction in short order.

But maybe there is a third possibility. Maybe . . . just maybe, the design of the body isn't faulty, and its inherent strength, the strength of the hunter-gatherer, remains in place. Maybe . . . just maybe, it doesn't need to be "fixed" with surgery or drugs when it "breaks."

I am convinced that there is no *maybe* about it. Nothing is wrong with the design; something is wrong with the *function*. It can be corrected and I'll show you how using the Egoscue Method.

2

Function Junction

If it walks like a duck, quacks like a duck, and keeps company with other ducks . . ." You know the rest of that old saw. It's another way of saying that form follows function. The duck looks like a duck because it's designed to quack and fly and do all the other things that ducks do.

I am being flippant because I am afraid this business about form and function tends to sound overly metaphysical. But one does not have to be a philosopher or a theologian to know that a design and its purpose are closely linked. A screwdriver looks the way it does because the tool's function is to drive screws. Violate the function and you violate the design. If the screwdriver is used as a crowbar or a chisel it will eventually break because such usages are not compatible with its design. And just like the screwdriver, the human body has a function that relates directly to its design; both must be in synchronization or the body will break.

One way to understand function as it applies to the body is to divide it into a couple of categories: 1) what we do with our bodies, and 2) what we don't do with our bodies.

Let's focus on what we don't do, first. In chapter one, I said that the body is a motion machine. I'll go one step further here: The body is a perpetual motion machine. From birth to death we are in constant motion. Our hearts beat, lungs expand and contract, individual cells surge and swirl. All of that, though, is involuntary. The machine is running on autopilot for those systems.

The musculoskeletal structure, however, is driven for the most part by our voluntary nervous system. Bear in mind this important point, though: Both systems interact and are interdependent. The voluntary side, by enervating the muscles which move the bones, energizes the involuntary systems; in turn, those sustain the voluntary functions by distributing oxygen and deploying white blood cells and making other vital contributions. If we eliminate the movement of either the voluntary or involuntary functions, both are imperiled.

We are, in fact, largely eliminating the movement of the musculoskeletal system every time we sit down in front of the TV set, climb behind the wheel of a car, or spend the work day at a desk. All of our other systems, dependent as they are on musculoskeletal motion, can't go it alone. They're not designed that way. The strain on those systems is enormous.

In short, we've got to move the body or we lose it.

SCI-FI COUCH POTATOES

Science-fiction writers have imagined a future peopled by a race of creatures with huge brains and shriveled bodies. It could happen, but I doubt it. Our bodies and minds live, prosper, and die together as a unit. For the most part, the learning curve generally corresponds to the life cycle's periods of growth and vigor. There are rare instances in which individuals' minds blossomed despite severe physical disability, but usually this surge of intellectual power kicks in after the physical development stage has had at least a chance to begin.

Once the body is deprived of the ability to move, extraordinary measures are necessary to keep its systems going. Sadly, it is a losing battle. What the sci-fi prophets forget about is that a shriveled body means shriveled and inadequate systems—respiratory, circulatory, digestive, immune, etc.

Although the subject of this chapter is the architecture of the body, a short detour is appropriate to examine one aspect of these motion-dependent systems. It will help illustrate my point about the interrelationships that are at work. When you ate breakfast this morning, your digestive system went to work. The toast and cereal eventually made their way through the small and large intestines. But how was that accomplished?

Gravity plays a big part in the digestive process; what goes in at the top comes out at the bottom. But gravity alone isn't enough. When you walk and run and bend and twist during the course of the day, breakfast is being pushed toward its final destination. The process is roughly 70 percent mechanical. The rest is attributable to chemistry, gravity, and diet.

Nutritionists are urging us to eat more fiber because it decreases what they call the "transit time" between intake and elimination, thereby reducing the risk of colon cancer. The quicker waste products are moved through the body, the less risk there is of toxic residues leaching out into the internal organs. But fiber, or lack of it, is just one element of the problem. Transit time increases as the body's movement decreases. It's one reason that physicians get their hospitalized patients out of bed as soon as possible.

There is mounting evidence that the high incidence of colon cancer in the United States is not exclusively a matter of diet. People of other nationalities, like the Argentines, consume more animal protein and fats than we do, yet their colon cancer rates are lower. This discrepancy is usually explained away as genetics or a result of eating onions or garlic or drinking a glass of wine with dinner.

Onions? How about motion? Those people haven't completely succumbed to the good life. They still walk. They rake leaves instead of using a blower. They swing an axe instead of firing up a chain saw. They wield a shovel, they don't ride a backhoe. For our part, we are not moving enough. As a result, our motion-dependent systems from digestive to circulatory, respiratory to immune, are breaking down.

REMEMBRANCE OF THINGS PAST

When we stop using a function it goes into a dormant state much like hibernation. Fortunately for us, the dysfunctional muscle doesn't slumber forever. It just waits patiently to be awakened and reminded of what it's really supposed to be doing. And that's the Egoscue Method's objective. We give the body a wake-up call in order to reacquaint it with its dormant functions. With a regular series of exercises, we say to the muscles "No, not that way—this way." In very short order, the body remembers, and function is restored.

Luckily, we never lose what's called the design sense. It's our kinesthetic sense that gets out of kilter. Basically, kinesthetic sense means a perception of the way we move. When I bend down to tie my shoe, I am activating certain muscles and bones. Since I practice what I preach, my design sense and kinesthetic sense are the same. The right nerves move the right muscles, which move the bones to the right places in the right sequence. But most people, depending on how dysfunctional they have become, are operating with major discrepancies between their design and kinesthetic senses. The right muscles are not moving the bones to the right places. The muscles of the low back, for instance, may have "forgotten" how to participate in the motion of tying a shoe, and the forgetfulness is compounded by weakness brought on by disuse.

The shoes get tied. The body is a master at improvisation. We'll squat down and our knees and thigh muscles will do most of the work. Or, from a sitting position the foot will be brought up and balanced on the opposite knee. When all else fails, there's always a pair of loafers.

I wish I knew why the design of the body allows a discrepancy to develop between the design sense and the kinesthetic sense. One possibility is that it foresees a situation in which a person could be deprived of motion, such as a long illness or injury. By allowing the design sense to be violated temporarily the body has the flexibility to survive these emergencies and eventually, when stability is restored, realign the design and kinesthetic senses.

What happens to modern man, though, is that the emergency never passes. We violate the design sense every minute of every hour of every day. By so doing, the body cannot operate according to design; the functions go into limbo and are never utilized again. This inevitably, and inexorably, leads to pain.

COMPENSATING MOTION

Even though we are not moving enough to maintain function, we are moving, and it is that motion—compensating motion—that causes the trouble. Muscles that were never intended to be involved in the walking, throwing, bending motions, to name three basic functions, are called into action to replace dysfunctional muscles. This puts stress and wear on the musculoskeletal system that it was not designed to handle. Like the screwdriver that's used as a crowbar, it breaks.

A functional muscle, for example, evenly distributes the shock transmitted into the sockets of the joint when the heel of the foot strikes the ground. But if there is dysfunction and compensation—the wrong muscle moving the bone into the wrong position—the shock is no longer evenly distributed; it's focused on one or two points in the socket and begins to wear away the cartilage.

Steve was one of approximately 1,500 patients I saw in 1990 with symptoms just like that. He was a runner who came into the clinic because of knee pain. Steve, like all my other patients, left his shoes in the waiting room when he came in for his first examination. We talked about running and his knees before I said "I'll bet the heel of your left shoe is worn more than the right." He admitted that his shoes wore unevenly, but couldn't remember which one took the worst beating.

"Why should one get chewed up faster than the other?" he asked. "Both feet are going around the track at the same time."

Steve went and got his shoes, and sure enough the left was definitely worn down further than the right. Steve was bearing most of his weight on the left side because of a dysfunctional right hip. By checking the right shoe I could observe a worn spot on the inside edge, evidence that the impact of the foot striking the ground was going nowhere near the tarsal area of the foot where it could be properly transmitted up the tibia and fibia to the knee.

We ignored Steve's knee. He did a half dozen exercises for his hip, shoulder, and head position, and he was running again without pain in about two weeks.

THE EYE OF THE BEHOLDER

Dysfunction is an observable condition. Back in chapter one I said the body sends us a message and a picture; I suppose you could call it an anatomical postcard. But we persist in misreading the postcard. One reason is that we've gotten so used to seeing the characteristics of dysfunction all around us that they look normal.

The worn spot in Steve's shoe seemed normal. Yesterday morning, when you drove to work, you probably saw dozens of people behind the steering wheels of other cars with their heads hanging forward and down from rounded shoulders. Didn't think twice about it, did you? All of those heads and shoulders looked perfectly normal; and all were perfectly dysfunctional. A highway full of people heading for work where sooner or later they'll experience symptoms of their dysfunctions—headaches, carpal tunnel, TMJ pain (an abbreviation for temporomandibular joint dysfunction, which affects the articulation of the lower jaw), etc.—and wonder why they feel so lousy.

Most people agree with everything I say about design and function. They examine the stick figure, take note of the right angles in the four socket position, marvel at the S-curve of the spine and then say, "But Pete, everybody's built a little different. This sloping right shoulder is just the way I'm put together." Or, "I look just the way my dad looked." All that means is that you have inherited Dad's environment, including its requisite motion or lack of motion, which produced the characteristic family shoulder. Everybody has the same design—that's what is inherited, not the rounded, dysfunctional shoulder.

What you're seeing in the mirror—and the time has come to stand in front of the mirror—is a reflection of your deviation from the design constant of the body.

Truly, what you see is what you get—function or dysfunction.

JUST A TWIST

We'll start at the bottom and work up. Your feet are designed to point straight ahead. Figure 5 illustrates the design constant for the foot. Notice that the feet are directly beneath the knees. The foot, in fact, goes where the hip and knee tell it to go. In the illustration, you can see the functional right angles that are formed.

In figure 6, the feet are cocked out or splayed like a duck. Look down at your feet. Are they straight ahead or splayed outward? Is one out and one straight? If the position of your feet resembles those in figure 6, you are violating the body's design.

"Well, I've always stood this way and don't feel any pain at all."

And maybe you never will—if you're lucky. But you'll never drive a golf ball correctly, for one thing. And there are dozens of

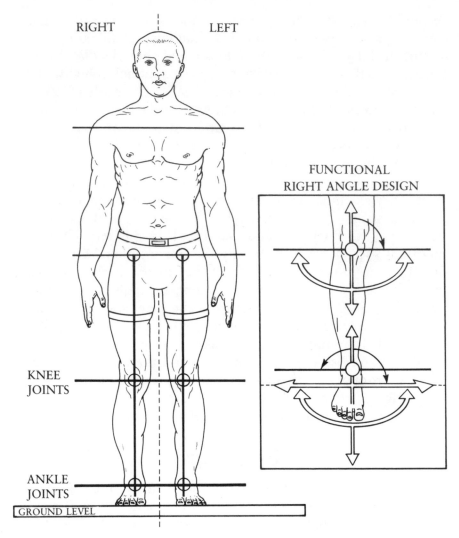

Figure 5
DESIGN CONSTANT OF THE FOOT

other sports and hundreds of routine, day-to-day activities that won't be accomplished as easily as they would if your kinesthetic and design senses coincided.

In figure 6, the feet are following orders. The gait muscles from the hip to the foot are in charge. Come up close to the mirror and examine your knees. Are the kneecaps pointing straight ahead or off to the left and/or right? Remember those right angles? The

RIGHT | LEFT

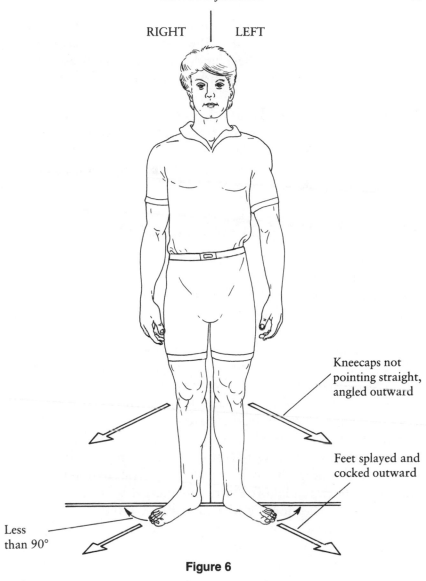

Kneecaps not
pointing straight,
angled outward

Feet splayed and
cocked outward

Less
than 90°

Figure 6

body fights to retain them. To do so, if your feet and knees are not pointing straight ahead, the body must introduce compensating motion when you walk.

The right angle articulation of the knee joint will occur, but at the same time there will be an outward-inward twisting movement to bring the foot down so that the body can move in a straight line. That lateral-medial twist is compensating motion.

This compensation is putting strain on the hip, knee, and ankle joints. The design gait motion of the foot—heel to toes, push off, heel to toes—changes to heel and toes working together as a platform, striking the ground either on the inside edge or the outside of the foot.

There's every likelihood that other kinds of compensating movement are going on at the same time, but if we consider nothing other than the outside-inside twisting movement of the knee, it becomes obvious that the extra motion, repeated hundreds, if not thousands, of times each day, is a ticking time bomb.

HEADED FOR TROUBLE

Next, stand back from the mirror and look at your hips. In figure 7, the model's hips are level, consistent with the body's design requirements of right angles and bifunctionality. In addition, his hips are square and sit directly under the shoulders and over the knees.

If you've distributed your weight evenly on both feet and the right hip is higher than the left (or vice versa), you are in violation of another design constant of the body. The penalty again is compensating motion, which is causing physical impairment right now, and will eventually lead to pain—if it hasn't already.

In the meantime, with a dysfunctional hip it is impossible to run, walk, or climb stairs efficiently. The same goes for bike riding, skating, and skiing. If nothing else, the dysfunctional hip will require you to expend more effort and energy. When someone tells me that he or she doesn't like to walk, I look at the hip and immediately know why. It takes too much effort to walk. They may have a million excuses—too busy, too rainy, too slippery, too dark and dangerous—but the real reason is that the dysfunctional hip is robbing them of the simple pleasure of going for a walk. And dysfunction leads to greater dysfunctions: "Walking? . . . I don't have time," becomes "I don't walk much anymore"; before long it's "I hate to walk," and finally "I can't walk."

The elevated hip that you may see in the mirror is affecting the normal gait pattern that allows us to walk in a straight line. If the gait pattern is functional, hip, knee, ankle, and foot move as a unit; there is smooth right-angle articulation of the joints; and

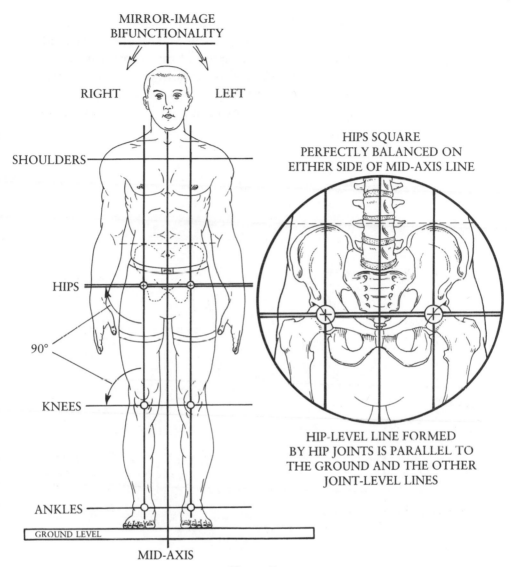

MIRROR-IMAGE
BIFUNCTIONALITY

RIGHT   LEFT

SHOULDERS

HIPS SQUARE
PERFECTLY BALANCED ON
EITHER SIDE OF MID-AXIS LINE

HIPS

90°

KNEES

HIP-LEVEL LINE FORMED
BY HIP JOINTS IS PARALLEL TO
THE GROUND AND THE OTHER
JOINT-LEVEL LINES

ANKLES

GROUND LEVEL

MID-AXIS

Figure 7

both sides of the body are doing exactly the same thing in a coordinated sequence. But if one hip is higher than the other (see figure 8), bifunctionality is affected. The muscles and bones on the high side are traveling farther and in a different direction in relation to the ground. As the leg swings free on the high side of the hip, the body is forced to tip toward the low side, and it produces stress in the knee and a waddling stride.

Often, discrepancies in the level of the hips mean that an individual is loading most of his weight on one side of the body. The body is compensating for the dysfunctional hip, sensing that it's doing something it's not supposed to be doing. Now the load-bearing side of the body is doing twice as much work as it was designed for. At the same time, the other hip is probably swinging

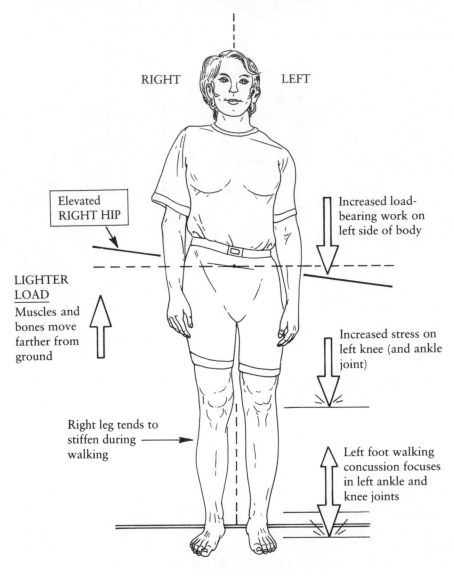

RIGHT   LEFT

Elevated
RIGHT HIP

Increased load-
bearing work on
left side of body

LIGHTER
LOAD
Muscles and
bones move
farther from
ground

Increased stress on
left knee (and ankle
joint)

Right leg tends to
stiffen during
walking

Left foot walking
concussion focuses
in left ankle and
knee joints

Figure 8

the right leg out in an arc because the leg muscles are not functioning according to the gait pattern. Hence, there's compensating motion in the hip joint; the leg is essentially stiff, with the hip doing the walking.

COMING AND GOING

Take another look at your hips. Does one hip seem to be a little closer to the mirror than the other? Figure 9 gives you an idea of what to look for. In addition to moving higher or lower, the hip can rotate to the right or left, and tilt forward or back. Another way to spot hip rotation is to sit down and relax. When you stand up again, look at your feet. If one foot is ahead of the other, it suggests that the hip on that side is moving forward.

Hip tilt may stand out more in profile by comparing one side of the body to the other. It would probably be a help to have someone take a photograph of you in profile. (We use a Polaroid camera in the clinic to save on processing time.)

In figure 10, the model's hips are both tilted forward. There is a reverse tilt in figure 11. If you think of hips as a three-foot-long shelf running parallel with the ground, the surface is actually tilting forward and back. Your belt line often reveals hip tilt. Seen from the side, a belt will angle forward or tip back, following the line of the tilt.

This hip tilt makes it harder for the body to maintain its right angles, which it must do. The tilt also interferes with bifunctionality because the muscles and the bones are not coming from, or going to, the same places on both sides of the body.

UNHINGED

Don't turn away from the mirror just yet. We still need to examine your shoulders. Again, the model's shoulders in figure 7 are level and parallel with the hips. Since the shoulders act as counterweights to the hips, and since the body is a unit, the shoulders react to the hips. An elevated right hip may mean an elevated right shoulder. But because of the way compensating motion can multiply and have numerous and different impacts throughout the unit, it's entirely possible to have an elevated right hip and a lowered right or elevated left shoulder. The combinations can be mixed and matched in many ways. But it doesn't really make any difference. As long as the shoulders are not level and parallel with the hips, the body's design is being violated.

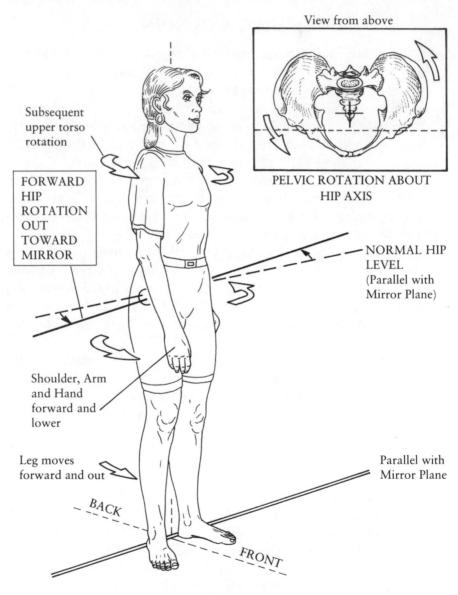

Subsequent upper torso rotation

FORWARD HIP ROTATION OUT TOWARD MIRROR

Shoulder, Arm and Hand forward and lower

Leg moves forward and out

BACK

FRONT

View from above

PELVIC ROTATION ABOUT HIP AXIS

NORMAL HIP LEVEL (Parallel with Mirror Plane)

Parallel with Mirror Plane

Figure 9

Our shoulders function with two different types of motion: ball and socket, like the hip, and a hinge, which provides a forward and back action. When we make rotations with our arms, as in a throwing motion, the ball and socket is used. The shoulder blades are part of this mechanism.

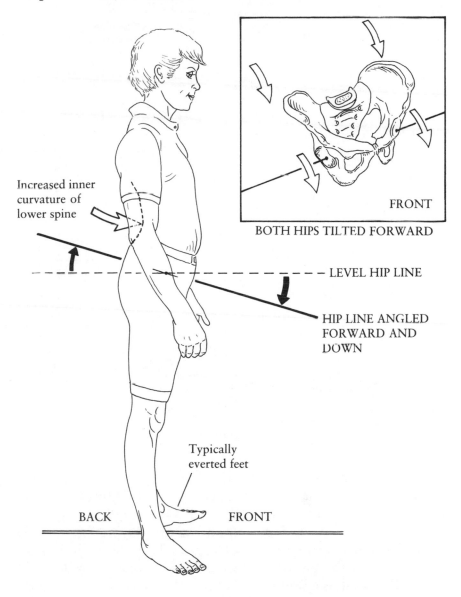

FRONT

BOTH HIPS TILTED FORWARD

Increased inner curvature of lower spine

LEVEL HIP LINE

HIP LINE ANGLED FORWARD AND DOWN

Typically everted feet

BACK   FRONT

Figure 10

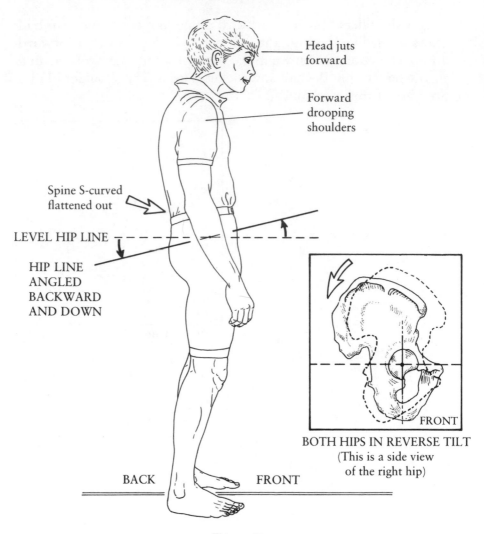

Head juts
forward

Forward
drooping
shoulders

Spine S-curved
flattened out

LEVEL HIP LINE

HIP LINE
ANGLED
BACKWARD
AND DOWN

FRONT

BOTH HIPS IN REVERSE TILT
(This is a side view
of the right hip)

BACK   FRONT

Figure 11

What does the elevated right shoulder in figure 12 tell us? Since the body is a unit, the shoulder is involved in the effort of hoisting up the stiff leg, which I referred to a few paragraphs ago, and flipping it into the walking position. Actors playing the role of a hunchback in a horror film walk like that. They throw the hip and leg forward with most of their weight on the opposite side of the body. The result is a shuffle and a lurch that make it seem as if the character is half paralyzed. Which in real life isn't far off the mark, minus the exaggeration and the theatrical flourishes.

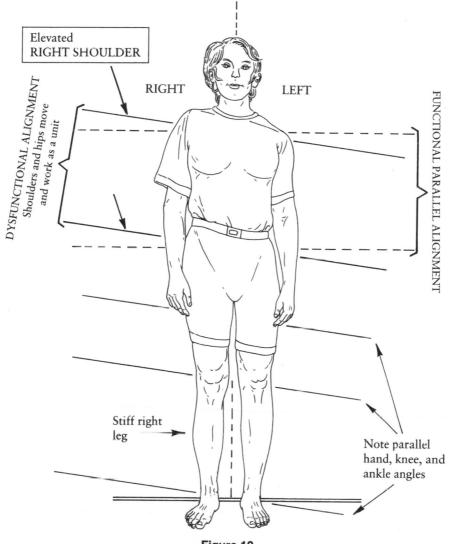

Elevated
RIGHT SHOULDER

RIGHT LEFT

DYSFUNCTIONAL ALIGNMENT
Shoulders and hips move
and work as a unit

FUNCTIONAL PARALLEL ALIGNMENT

Stiff right
leg

Note parallel
hand, knee, and
ankle angles

Figure 12

UNCOMMONLY COMMON

A side view of your shoulders may also show that they are rolled
forward. The stooped shouldered look is very common (see figure
13). The hinge joint allows the shoulders to come forward, and
they stay in that position because we are not bearing our weight
in the functional, four socket position, with the head, shoulders,
hips, knees, and ankles in line.

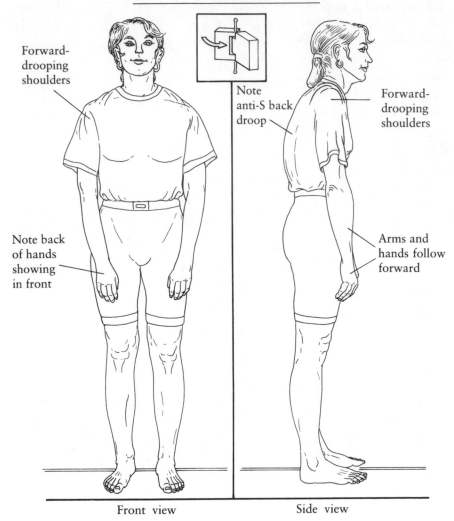

Each shoulder's hinge joint
"locks" shoulder forward
due to dysfunctional weight bearing

Forward-
drooping
shoulders

Note
anti-S back
droop

Forward-
drooping
shoulders

Note back
of hands
showing
in front

Arms and
hands follow
forward

Front view

Side view

Figure 13
STOOPED SHOULDERS ROLLED FORWARD

Once the shoulders get locked into the forward hinge position, the shoulder blades and the rest of the shoulder mechanism are immobilized. Rotator cuff problems (involving a group of four muscles located near the deltoid muscle near the shoulder blade) used to be rare. Today, the orthopedic surgeons are kept busy fixing rotator cuffs.

What's being fixed is this: There's usually stiffness in the shoulder or the vicinity of the shoulder blade, pain, ranging from dull aches to sharp jabs, and restricted movement of the arm. The real source of the problem lies elsewhere: the rounded shoulder that is being asked to make ball-and-socket motions at the same time it is locked into the forward-hinged position. With the shoulder forward, the rotator cuff muscles are unable to assist in the abduction of the arm because they are being prevented from rotating the head of the humerus bone the way they're supposed to. It's similar to breaking a key off in a lock. If the rotator cuff is forced hard enough—whacking a tennis ball, a golf ball, a baseball can do it—the muscles will tear.

Typically, surgeons go in and repair the damage or, in some cases, shave down the head of the humerus to remove the "obstruction."

A HEAVY LOAD

You may have noticed the position of your head while you were checking out your shoulders in the mirror (see figure 14). Dysfunctional shoulder and back muscles can hardly be expected to hold the head in an upright position. That's a lot of work. The head is heavy and balanced on top of the spinal column. But even if they wanted to—and they do want to—the muscles can't allow the head to flop forward and down. Thus, dysfunctional or not, the muscles are under great strain.

Drop your chin toward your chest and you'll feel a tightness across the top of your upper back. The "echo" of that tightness reverberates all the way to the hip. The muscles in your upper torso are fighting to keep you in an upright position and it's a losing battle. Back spasms, neck aches, migraine headaches, excruciating jaw pain, dizziness, blurred vision are all indications of how hard the body is struggling to stay upright.

The head is very sensitive to movement and position. The flow of blood and oxygen is all uphill, and it doesn't help matters when the upper torso is dysfunctional and under strain. Watch a demoralized, losing team on a ball field. You'll see sagging shoulders and drooping heads. The poor performance is reflected in the postures. Which came first, the poor posture or the poor performance? The form or the (dys)function? And now we're right back

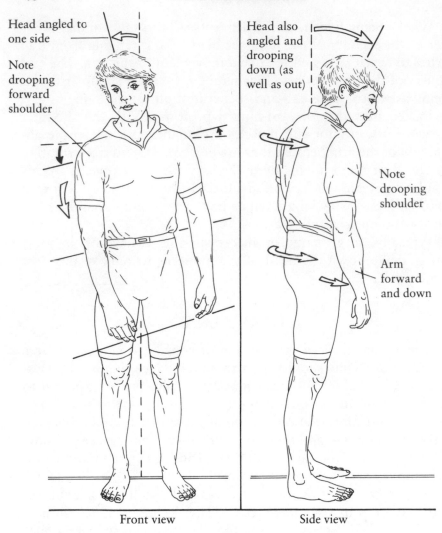

Head angled to
one side

Note
drooping
forward
shoulder

Head also
angled and
drooping
down (as
well as out)

Note
drooping
shoulder

Arm
forward
and down

Front view   Side view

Figure 14

to the cosmic theme that opened the chapter. But this isn't meta-physics; it's health, fitness—life.

Why are we hurting? Why are we losing our competitive edge? Why are so many of us stressed out, depressed, angry, and unfulfilled?

Perhaps this incident will help provide answers. A few years ago, a major league baseball pitcher came into my clinic. He was twenty-eight years old at the time. I'll call him Bill, though that wasn't his name. He was suffering from chronic, severe back spasms; his control was gone and it looked like Bill's career was over. On top of the physical problem, he was profoundly depressed. On his first visit Bill told me he was considering suicide.

The strategy I decided to use with him works with intensely competitive people. I set out to make Bill angry with me. In effect, I told him he was a coward, knowing that a coward would never have made it onto a major league pitcher's mound. After getting him "torqued," I began the therapeutic process. Within a half hour Bill's pain was gone, and by the time he left the clinic the depression had also lifted.

Why? By performing several basic exercises, Bill was getting his body back into its design form. Immediately, the functions that had become dysfunctional reacted. His spirits improved along with the functions. Bill was simply feeling better for the first time in months, probably in years. His sense of well-being began to return as his body moved closer to its true design. Today he's back in action and there's no more talk of suicide.

The body "stays in touch." Pain is one form of communication. But important messages are not always delivered in a shout or a shriek. Sometimes the body whispers to us; we hear it and we're afraid. But no matter how it arrives, the message is of vital importance.

I think of Bill and his depression whenever I read about chronic fatigue syndrome, which has been rather unkindly nicknamed "yuppie flu." I've seen recent reports that say 2 to 5 million Americans have had the symptoms: fever, lymph node swelling, diarrhea, mood swings, and panic attacks.

What's going on here?

Before we conclude that humankind is facing a new disease, we should first take another look in the mirror.

3

The Two R's — Relevance and Responsibility

Most fitness and physical therapy programs run into trouble because an important fact of life gets overlooked. Humans only do what gives them pleasure. In terms of motivational concepts, it doesn't come any simpler. We climb mountains because we like the thrill, run marathons because we thrive on challenge, work eighty hours a week because we crave money or prestige or responsibility.

Pleasure can be fatiguing, dangerous, painful. But it is still pleasure. We needed Sigmund Freud to come along and give it a name, but the United States is founded on the "pleasure principle"—the pursuit of happiness. The words are in the Declaration of Independence. And we pursue happiness with every waking hour.

Let's use this chapter to explore the implications of the pleasure principle. I believe it will explain why we have come to a standstill after ten thousand years of pursuing our pleasure and our survival one step at a time.

A BELLY FULL

A vital connection, the one that links pleasure and motion, has been broken. When primitive man, the hunter-gatherer, spent the day tracking a herd of elk, he probably was not conscious of a feeling of pleasure. He didn't stop at midday, look down at the calluses on his bare feet and say, "Gosh, this is fun!" The pleasure came after the kill when he got back to the village and filled his belly with elk meat.

The next day at dawn he returned to the hunt. Why? He liked

eating. There was a cause and effect relationship that linked motion and survival and pleasure.

Perhaps humans learned this lesson the hard way. Sitting around the village telling tall elk stories was undoubtedly more enjoyable than trudging across the tundra on a cold day. Those who succumbed to the temptation soon found that their food supply was dwindling. Short rations meant that glucose levels in the bloodstream declined and there was a resulting loss of energy. The hunter's stamina and eye-hand coordination deteriorated. Soon, there was hunger, starvation, and death.

The experience taught the survivors that the motion associated with hunting or gathering was not optional. It was a necessity of life. Any pleasure that came to them—a meal, a feast day, the warmth of a fire—was the direct result of movement. The idea was so basic that it wasn't an idea at all. Pure instinct drove our ancestors to move, and the body's design and function operated in tandem.

LACK OF MOTION AND SOCIAL STATUS

Are there two activities more movement-intense than working and playing? If, in a word association game, I said "work," the comeback could well be "shovel" or "sweat." However, work is done sitting down for most of us. The prelude to work is commuting—more sitting in a car, train, or bus. Even our playtime, recreation, lacks motion. We watch sports on TV, take a drive into the country, curl up with a good book.

In many ways, movement is now associated with drudgery and not pleasure. Most Americans aspire to white collar jobs. Professional and social status tends to be determined along the dividing line between those who perform physical labor and those who don't. Our educational and social system has reinforced that bias.

Additionally, at home, this has been the century of labor-saving appliances. In the kitchen and elsewhere around the house, our grandmothers moved their upper torsos—particularly arms and shoulders—through a full range of motion as they chopped and kneaded and stirred, hung wash out to dry, cleaned windows, and beat dusty carpets. Today, the instant gourmet opens a package and flicks the switch of a food processor. In many households the simple chore of sweeping the floor is performed by an "electric broom," or vacuum cleaner. Outside in the backyard, grass clippers that required bending at the waist, as well as hand, wrist, elbow, and shoulder involvement, have given way to gasoline powered string-trimmers. Old wooden-handled hedge shears, requiring a good workout of the rotator cuff muscles, have gone all-electric, and a muscle-powered hand mower is an oddity. Once these outdoor chores are performed, the "zapper" or remote control device makes it possible to spend the rest of the day watching television without stirring off the sofa to change the channel. And what a major effort it seems to be when the "zapper" is broken and we have to change channels the old-fashioned way!

The purpose of all these gadgets, aside from enriching their inventors and manufacturers, is to free us from time-consuming, "backbreaking" tasks. And there's nothing wrong with that; the name of the game is the pursuit of pleasure, after all. But liberation has led to a new form of slavery. We are virtually shackled to inanimate objects. They don't move, and we don't move.

THE USUAL SUSPECTS

The three-way alliance of motion, design, and function depends on a very crude glue to bind it together: reward and punishment. The problem with what's going on in our culture now is that there is no longer an overt penalty for loss of design-function. Once, if you couldn't kill the elk, couldn't catch him, couldn't throw straight—you and your clan died out. The ultimate penalty. You paid for being a lousy or lazy hunter. Survival of the fittest. But these days there doesn't *seem* to be an overt penalty.

But what seems to be is often not what is. Though it may be delayed, there is a penalty, usually a penalty of pain or dysfunction, rather than immediate extinction. Furthermore, the pain does not appear to be chronic. It *seems* initially to be an episodic event.

MISTAKEN IDENTITY

The generic problem is one of relevance. Motion seems to be irrelevant to our day-to-day lives. We don't raise our hands over our heads because we don't have to. Our shoulders stay hinged forward because we don't need to throw a rock or spear accurately. Being eaten by the tiger or bludgeoned by the guy from the next valley who wants to steal the cattle provide immediate readouts on dysfunctional shoulders. But months elapse, even years, before a wrist starts to hurt—the punishment for a dysfunctional shoulder—and then we blame it on a word processor's keyboard.

Instead of making the connection between the pain and lack of motion, we round up the usual suspects: arthritis, tennis elbow, carpal tunnel syndrome. The misguided search for relevance leads us to concoct cause and effect relationships that don't exist. "My back hurts . . . I'm going to get a better pair of running shoes." "If these neck aches don't go away, I'm going to cut down on my reading to an hour a day."

Now, there's the ultimate in mistaken identity. Reading. We've become so dysfunctional that the act of sitting in a chair and reading is presumed to be too much of a strain on the neck and back muscles. And the remedy is to do less reading—or less running, walking, skiing. We restrict our movements because we start to think that movement itself is the problem.

Eventually, dysfunction breeds dysfunction until all the motion-dependent systems of the body are affected: Can't sleep, can't eat, can't walk, can't breathe.

SILENT PARTNERS

There are many definitions of fitness. Here's mine: The positive control of one's environment on a daily basis without effort. What's the point of all those sit-ups and bench presses, the fish oil and oat bran, the diets and the jogging, if we cannot control our personal environment in a way that fulfills our physical and psychological needs?

It's not as complicated as it might seem on first reading. By *environment* I mean the small envelope of space that a person inhabits at any given moment: the bedroom, the office, the backyard, the putting green at the country club. Control at this level, as modest as it is in scope, constitutes the source of our sense of well-being.

As for the other elements of my definition of fitness—control and effort—think in terms of a successful business executive who, to maximize his use of wasted commuting time, hires a driver and installs a cellular phone in the car. He is controlling his environment without effort. On the other hand, if the executive's career takes a bad turn and he can't afford the phone or the driver, he is in danger of losing control. The guy doesn't give up without a fight, though. He speeds around the traffic jams by using the emergency lane, he reads and drives at the same time, and works an extra two hours a day. Effort. So much effort that he ends up having a heart attack.

But before a health crisis, like a heart attack or an agonizing back spasm, occurs, the body tells us we are starting to lose control. There's a common physician's rule of thumb that when an individual becomes aware of an internal organ, angina pain or kidney pain, for instance, then there is a problem with that organ. The same goes for muscles and bones; and it applies to the accoutrements of everyday life that we take for granted. When the toaster starts to buzz and smoke, it's not a bad idea to pull the plug. Therefore, if, in the normal course of living, working, and playing, we start hearing from our silent partners, it is time for us to listen to what they are saying: "You have lost positive control of your personal environment on a daily basis without effort."

Sure, anybody who hasn't jogged in years is going to huff and puff after giving in to the impulse to run around the block. But if it is an effort to climb the front stairs without breathing heavily, or if we get leg cramps after an hour of driving, or feel listless most of the time, or anxious, or angry, then something is wrong. If I call in sick because I can't stand the back pain from sitting in my desk chair for another day, then clearly I am not, by definition, fit—no matter how often I visit the health club.

IS THE MEDIUM THE MESSAGE?

The body is using the leg cramps or the shortness of breath to deliver a message. But we've developed a tin ear when it comes to listening to the body. I think it's because of the pleasure principle that I mentioned earlier. The body is saying "Move!" The pleasure principle comes back with, "Move? Moving hurts . . . forget it." And by assuming that motion is not relevant, it's all that much easier to give up, and a small bit of control over the personal environment is also relinquished.

Unlike the type-A business executive who ran himself ragged trying to retain control, responsibility for fitness and function is all too often given up without much of a fight. We don't even realize that we're losing it. There is a gradual attrition that takes place over time that is camouflaged by modern technology. For one thing, the *sturm und drang* of the workplace convinces us that we are in constant motion. "Boy, am I tired. I think I'll take a sleeping pill to make sure I get enough rest tonight."

And I hear comments like that all the time. Patients come into the clinic complaining about insomnia, and when we investigate their daily physical routines, it becomes obvious why they need pills to sleep: Their bodies aren't tired at the end of the day. Why? The patients hardly move at all from 9:00 A.M. to 5:00 P.M. When I point that out, the response is "I take a mental pounding every day." And they probably do. But by refusing to go to sleep, the body—not the mind—is saying "I haven't done a lick of work."

Television is also good at convincing us that we're moving when we're sitting still; in control when there is no control. It promises "You Are There," and "Be There!" But we don't have to budge off the couch. We seem to be able to directly participate in events without moving. Again, motion doesn't seem relevant.

By this point I hope I've demonstrated how wrong that is. It's time to reintroduce the other R-word.

Responsibility.

We have about 10,000 clinical visits a year at my clinic in San Diego. Many of the patients are in pain. Some come in because they're not satisfied with their health or level of fitness. Others are trying to master a sport, a recreational activity, or a profession. While their motives are different, in almost every case there is one starting point. By the time those people walk through the front door and into our reception area, they are instinctively ready to take responsibility for their health.

That is the essential ingredient, yet it's the hardest thing for many people to come to terms with, and the reason is deeply rooted in our consumer society. We are surrounded by products. It's a twentieth century phenomenon. I don't want to get into sociology, but this consumer mindset, which is conditioned to believe that nearly anything is available for the right price, is at odds with the need to take responsibility for our own health.

Health is not a product.

Yet many of us come at health care with the reflexes and values of a hardened veteran of the shopping mall wars. Like the insomniac who purchases sleep off the drug store shelf, rather than going for a brisk walk after dinner, there is an over-reliance on a host of medical procedures that should be reserved for "last resort" situations. It's become second nature to try and buy our way out of an illness with surgery or medication when the only effective way out is to take responsibility and alter a self-destructive lifestyle.

I see hundreds of patients each year who have either undergone joint replacement surgery or are considering it. With the exception of accident victims, whose joints have been destroyed—and I mean destroyed, not banged around—there hasn't been a single case that wouldn't have been better off with a less traumatic, alternative treatment.

But artificial knees and hips and shoulder joints are state-of-the-art medicine with high price tags, and therefore seem to have more cachet and credibility than going back to the basic design of the body, restoring lost functions, and maintaining them with a half hour of exercises each day.

MR. GOODWRENCH AND THE BODY

Another questionable assumption is that we can "fix" the body the way we fix a car by replacing the flat tire or doing a brake job. The neighborhood mechanic hears a rattle, finds the defective part, unscrews a few bolts, attaches a replacement, and we drive off. The process seems so simple and straightforward that modern physicians have adopted the same methodology. The shoulder hurts: Remove the appropriate joint and bolt on another.

Breathtaking technological advances have allowed us to treat the human body like a Toyota Corolla. A hundred years ago, we didn't have the tools or the material. Today, both are available and, as a rule, man uses his inventions and new-found capabilities for the simple reason that they are there to be used. The consequences and ramifications of the use are left to be sorted out at a later date.

In the rush to embrace new technology, physicians have forgotten the basic anatomical lesson that their predecessors observed by default. A hundred years ago there was no way physicians could change the body's design even if they wanted to. But they also kept faith with the body's design by inclination. A country doctor knew, without giving the idea a second thought, that there was nothing wrong with the design. He could see his patients using their bodies to bring in the hay and split kindling. When accidents struck, he strapped on a splint and waited for the body's natural healing power to take its course. In the 1990s, we think we're a lot smarter than the country doctor—so smart that we know the body is too frail to withstand the punishing onslaught of a desk chair without the benefit of drugs, surgery, or machines.

A PRESIDENTIAL PAIN

I was a Marine combat officer in Vietnam. One evening a Vietcong with an AK-47 bought me a ticket on a medevac chopper. Marine aviators—the grunts called them "airedales"—brought the helicopter into a hillside landing zone after dark, sliding the ship in sideways under the trees. The late VC's buddies—he was late a half second after pulling the trigger—gave me a rousing sendoff.

That's my first and last war story, and I'm telling it as a way to acknowledge that I know how stressful pain can be. I understand how someone wants the pain to go away and to go away now. But what I can't understand is the attitude, not driven by pain, that says "Okay, replace the hip if you think it's necessary."

Gerald R. Ford is a case in point. In 1990, I was asked to consult with the former president, who was considering knee replacement surgery. I went out to Palm Springs, California to visit with Mr. Ford at his home. He was swimming, exercising, and golfing. For a guy with a "bad" knee, he was leading a very active life.

You may remember the picture of President Ford tumbling down the stairs of Air Force One in Salzburg, Austria. Chevy Chase, one of the comedians on "Saturday Night Live," had a field day with that one. To keep the boss from looking like a klutz, his press secretary put out the word that the fall was caused by a knee problem dating back to Ford's days as a college football player.

But what I saw in Palm Springs was a hip, a knee, and a foot dysfunction that probably predated the University of Michigan and Yale (where Ford coached the freshman football team and attended law school). The right foot was splayed outward and the right hip was elevated. Over the years, the knee, caught in the middle of a tug-of-war, had lost most of its cartilage. The football injury was an early symptom of the dysfunction. By putting the joint's right angles under stress and then falling on it, or being hit by a 200-pound linesman, the knee was strained beyond the breaking point.

In Mr. Ford's case, a common mistake was made. There were two overlapping cause and effect relationships at work, and one was being ignored.

There was a presumption that football damaged President Ford's knee. It seems perfectly logical if you accept the idea that football is dangerous, and accidents do happen when hefty young men are allowed to spend an afternoon crashing into each other. But why did Mr. Ford get hurt when three (or four or five, the exact number isn't important) of his teammates, the same basic size, just as gutsy and hard-driving, played an entire season—or several—without incident? Luck?

Not luck. Unlike his uninjured teammates, Ford was an accident waiting to happen. A unique and personal set of environmental conditions (the cause) restricted his range of motions until dysfunctions set in (the effect). Years later, cause and effect no. 2 occurred on the fifty-yard line.

The stretcher bearers carried young Jerry Ford off the field. The doctors fixed what was broken. But the repair work didn't take the dysfunction into account. Gradually, the impact of walking and skiing on a dysfunction that wasn't evenly spreading the pressure around in the knee joint took its toll by scraping the cartilage away.

Next stop Salzburg.

However embarrassed President Ford might have been, he wasn't in pain. And when I saw him about fifteen years later, the primary complaint about his knees (notice that we've gone from knee singular to knees plural) was that a feeling of weakness would occur when he was trying to hit a golf ball out of a sand trap.

The weakness in the knees was a symptom of cartilage loss, and that, in turn, was a symptom of a hip dysfunction that Mr. Ford had not recognized until I pointed it out to him. Let me explain a few things about cartilage before we go any further. There is nothing very complex or mysterious about it. There are three types—hyaline, elastic, and fibrous. Basically it is a connective tissue similar to a chewy piece of gristle in an otherwise tender sirloin steak.

Most of the skeleton in early fetal stages is comprised of cartilage; as the fetus develops, a hard matrix of mineralized ground substance, collagen fiber, and embedded cells replaces the cartilage, leaving small amounts of the original "gristle" at the ends of the bones. This type of cartilage, hyaline, acts as a shock absorber and buffer when bone comes into contact with bone. In addition, we all have some elastic cartilage in our noses, ears, and windpipes. That's where the flexibility comes from in those organs. The disks, or menisci, of the vertebrae are fibrous cartilage.

Research has shown that hyaline cartilage will swell by 12 or 13 percent during warm-up exercises, making the joints more capable of withstanding stress. Furthermore, extended physical training, particularly running, enlarges the cartilage cells and increases their metabolic activity. The collagen fiber in the disks of the vertebrae also increase when the back is under sustained pressure.

I gave Mr. Ford a series of exercises to reintroduce movement and restore the lost functions, and he did them faithfully for several weeks. On my follow-up visit, I asked him if the exercises were getting easier to do. He said they were—but . . .

"But what?" I inquired.

"The knees aren't improving," he said.

Gerald Ford had just gotten through telling me that the exercises were easier to do than when he first started, a clear indication that the knees were stronger and more functional, which is what I went on to explain to him.

Mr. Ford listened and nodded his head as I ran through the anatomical principles involved. In the end, the former president said he understood but that since an operation was scheduled he thought he would just go ahead and have a knee replaced anyway.

I asked again if there was pain.

"No, they're not hurting," he said.

I was totally baffled, totally frustrated. Here was a guy who was willing to take responsibility for his health: He did the exercises every day without fail. He was making real progress. Yet it made more sense to him to throw his knee away and buy a new one.

Someone had assured President Ford that the cartilage was "gone" in his knees. I told him that the body is not given a fixed amount of cartilage that is used up and never replaced.

"If you give it a chance the body will replace the cartilage that has been scraped away," I said. We grow hair and fingernails; a damaged heart can spontaneously bypass an arterial blockage; millions of new cells are created each day.

The only reason for thinking that cartilage is permanently lost is that the dysfunction that wears away the tissue in the first place is allowed to be permanent. The cartilage does not regenerate because it is being worn down faster than it is being built up.

Early in 1992, Gerald Ford had the other knee replaced, and both are now operating with the old dysfunction. To understand what's going on inside the former president's knees, make one hand into a fist, and smack the fist into the palm of your other hand. Concave and convex surfaces are coming together, much like a golf ball sitting on top of a tee. First, exert even and steady pressure with the fist. Now, roll the knuckles of the first downward and push. The result is a noticeable pressure point instead of a smooth distribution of the force.

By smacking your fist into the hand, with the knuckles taking the brunt of the impact, and twisting, you have duplicated the action of Mr. Ford's dysfunctional knees. He is in his seventies, and any doctor who installed the artificial joints in a man of his age would probably figure that even with the pressure point the devices will outlast the rest of the body (and there's no cartilage to wear away). But what about the ball and socket just up the line, the one in the hip? An avid golfer, President Ford will put the new knees through their paces. There will be no feeling of weakness when he hits out of sand traps.

Heads up!

All that new-found snap, crackle, and pop that hadn't been going into the "bad" knees also wasn't going into the hip. Now, by using his state-of-the-art knees, like his knees haven't been used in years, the dysfunction is working all that much harder on the hips.

When Gerald Ford's back starts to hurt, he will chalk it up to age, telling his golfing buddies all the while that the smartest thing he ever did was to have knee replacement surgery.

4

Self-Diagnosis

What we've done so far amounts to the initial stages of planning a journey. The first thing was to decide on the destination. Well, we know where we're going and why. The next step is to draw a map.

Diagnosis is the starting point. I group function-dysfunction into four categories, or conditions. Conditions I, II, and III are clusters of dysfunctional symptoms. They are easy to recognize, and by the end of this chapter you'll find yourself doing a mental diagnosis on just about everyone you encounter.

The fourth category really isn't a condition, since the term implies dysfunction. I call it "D-lux." The "D" is for design. Occasionally, very occasionally, you'll spot a real live D-lux, a person with all of his or her right angles and horizontal lines—picture perfect and posture perfect! My goal is to get every reader of this book into the D-lux category.

In chapter two, I had you stand in front of a mirror and take a good long look. If you saw a body with all of its right angles, head back, level and in line with the shoulders, both shoulders level and over the hips, hips square and parallel with the knees, knees pointing straight ahead and over the feet, and feet aimed straight ahead—if that's what you saw—look again.

You may be a member of the privileged D-lux minority, the truly functional, and I hope that's the case. Or, more likely, your eye is being deceived, which easily happens because we're so accustomed to looking at dysfunction. Imagine that I have drawn a series of parallel lines on your mirror. In fact, you might find it helpful to do that yourself, using masking tape and a carpenter's level. Horizontally, there should be four lines running left to right through your shoulder, hip, knee, and ankle joints. Vertically, two lines connect the shoulder to the hip to knee to the foot. The result is a grid just like the one shown in figure 1 (see page 7). A series of right angles form where the lines intersect at the joints.

To help you visualize the body's right-angle design, adjust the waistband of your shorts or trousers while standing in front of the mirror. Pull the right side up higher than the hip, and slide the other side below the left hip. The line formed by the waistband goes off at an angle. It's not parallel with your shoulders.

Next, you'll need to readjust the waistband to make it run from hip to hip. If your tummy sticks out, the line will be bowed, but the right and left ends of it should be on the same plane—that is, if you're functional.

Now check the line of your hips with the line of your shoulders. Functional hips and shoulders will be parallel. Are yours? Or do the lines diverge or converge, as they do in figures 8 and 12 (pages 32, 37)?

Don't try to adjust your lines. Just stand there and relax. Let the body fall into its natural position. One of the reasons that the hundreds of books that have been published on back pain ultimately fail is that they tell you to stand up straight, or to keep your knees bent slightly while shaving or brushing your teeth. A dysfunctional body will do its own dysfunctional thing no matter what instructions we give it.

Okay. Lines still parallel? If they are, bravo: You are D-lux. I have no interest in convincing you that I'm right and you're wrong when it comes to your own body. It's a mistake to try to superimpose my "expert opinion" on your judgment. I'm not the expert: You are. I can browbeat anybody into looking and looking until they finally see what I want them to see. But in the end, they don't really see anything at all.

Just an additional word of advice, though. The eye is easy to fool. Every now and then I'll have a patient who just cannot see his or her own dysfunctions. Linda is a prime example. She could see that her feet were everted, that her toes turned outward (eversion tips the pelvis forward, inversion tips it to the rear), but she didn't notice her elevated hip or shoulder.

We were in my office and she was sitting in front of the desk in an arm chair with a low back. I said to her, "You don't like my chair, do you?"

"No, it's fine, really."

"Why are you fidgeting around then?"

"I guess I'm just a fidgety person," she said with shrug.

"I've had those chairs specially designed to tell me a few things about my patients. I'm going to write a note to myself predicting how you'll answer the next question I ask you." I stopped and wrote the note. "Okay, where's all the weight being supported as you sit in that chair? Is it on the right buttock or the left?"

Linda thought about it. Fidgeted a little more and said, "The left."

I smiled and held up the note pad for her to see. I had written, "left."

I explained to Linda that while she couldn't see her dysfunctional right hip, she could feel it. The weight on her left side was symptomatic of the dysfunction. Weight should be supported equally on both sides. Linda's right hip couldn't take the burden because it was out of position, and she was having spasms of the low back.

So if you can't see the symptoms of conditions I, II, and III, try to feel them. Weight distribution is one thing to check, another is whether one hip or shoulder feels tighter (or looser) than the other. Is it easier to back the car down the driveway looking over your right or left shoulder? There shouldn't be any difference. If there is, it's a symptom of dysfunction.

Even after you've looked and felt, and if all your right angles are there, keep reading. This chapter will give you diagnostic tools that will be of use to the members of your family, friends, and co-workers. The section that deals with the D-lux category at the end of this chapter will explain more about it and you will find maintenance exercises in chapter five. If you are really D-lux, the challenge is to stay there in spite of today's sedentary lifestyle.

A final comment for readers who are in pain: I don't believe in being macho about pain. It must not be ignored. Before reading further in this chapter, turn ahead to chapter five and take a look at the section on pain suppression (pages 82–83). But don't get sidetracked. Come back here and finish the self-diagnosis. I've said it before, and I'll say it again—pain is not your problem. Pain is a symptom of the problem.

Condition I

I've included drawings based on pictures from my clinic's files of people whose hips and shoulders are out of "true," as carpenters would say about warped two-by-fours. In figures 15, 16, and 17 you are seeing individuals who are not at all unusual in terms of their dysfunctions.

What I am looking for initially is Condition I: hips tilted forward, feet everted (figure 15).

Your waistband will be of help again. Imagine looking at a two-six-pack-a-day man. The beer has given him a large gut, which hangs over his belt. Seen from the side, it looks like a shelf slowly collapsing under the weight of all that flab, the leading edge flaring down and away at a 10- or 15-degree angle. If your waistband is headed in that same direction, it indicates that your pelvis is tilted forward. The beer belly look is not only a reflection of a large thirst, it develops because dysfunctional men in general exhibit a forward tilt to the pelvis. The beer may produce the paunch, but that distinctive angle comes from the pelvis. Traditionally, we're more likely to see a pelvis tilted *under* in women, for reasons I will explain as we proceed.

If you turn sideways to the mirror, the angle of the pelvis may be even more obvious, as in figure 16. To understand hip tilt, put your hands in front of you, palms down, elbows bent at 90 degrees. Interlock the fingers as if you were about to crack your knuckles. Next, roll your hands slightly so that the palms come toward your stomach or chest. The backs of the hands form a shelf similar to the pelvis, and that pelvic shelf is tipping forward, allowing the belly to slide down and away. One way to think of it is that a restaurant's pastry cart has gotten loose and is rolling down a set of stairs with pies and cakes and mousse tumbling off the front.

Pelvic tilt is the source of much of the minor low back pain that many of us take for granted as we get into our thirties and forties. By increasing the arch of the spine, this dysfunction is like a hairline crack in the wall of a dam. The overall structure is weakened. In time the crack gets wider. The constant flexion of the

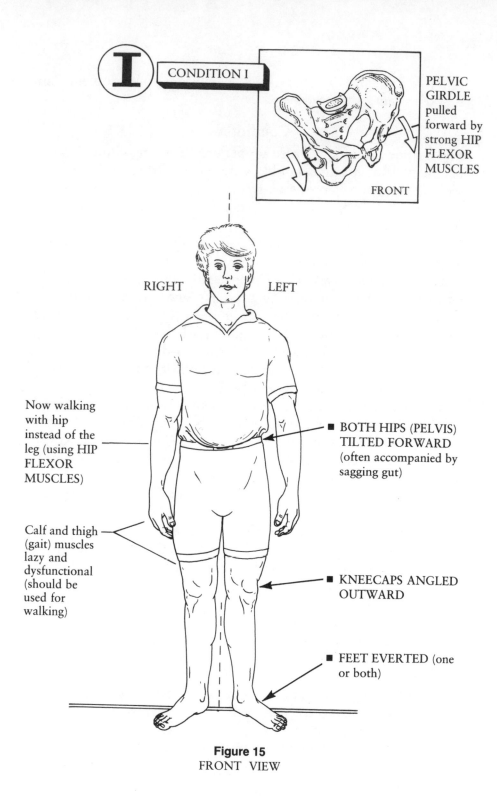

CONDITION I

PELVIC GIRDLE pulled forward by strong HIP FLEXOR MUSCLES

FRONT

RIGHT   LEFT

Now walking with hip instead of the leg (using HIP FLEXOR MUSCLES)

Calf and thigh (gait) muscles lazy and dysfunctional (should be used for walking)

■ BOTH HIPS (PELVIS) TILTED FORWARD (often accompanied by sagging gut)

■ KNEECAPS ANGLED OUTWARD

■ FEET EVERTED (one or both)

Figure 15
FRONT VIEW

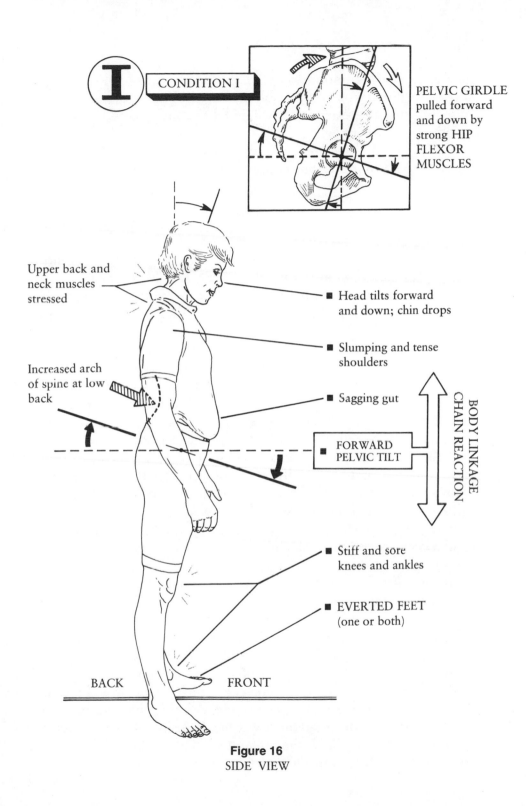

CONDITION I

PELVIC GIRDLE pulled forward and down by strong HIP FLEXOR MUSCLES

Upper back and neck muscles stressed

Head tilts forward and down; chin drops

Slumping and tense shoulders

Increased arch of spine at low back

Sagging gut

FORWARD PELVIC TILT

BODY LINKAGE CHAIN REACTION

Stiff and sore knees and ankles

EVERTED FEET (one or both)

BACK   FRONT

Figure 16
SIDE VIEW

spine, beyond its normal range, is putting wear and tear on the vertebral disks. You've probably heard of "lumbago," or "sciatica," which is the result of a herniated disk causing compression of a spinal nerve root.

As far as I'm concerned hip tilt is worth treating before it develops into a more serious condition.

EVERSION

You've just tackled the hard part of the diagnosis for Condition I. Everted feet are easy to spot. Stand the way you normally would. Shift your feet around, move them back and forth, let them go where they want to go. If you see a V-shape, your heels forming the apex, one foot going to the right, the other to the left, you're looking at eversion.

The situation is the rough equivalent of having two flat tires. The big gait muscles of the legs have stopped working. Everted feet mean you are walking with your hips. The feet evert because the gait muscles have become lazy and transferred the walking function to the hip flexor muscles. If I shot a slow-motion video tape of a functional foot and leg in the act of walking, we would see the heel strike the ground, the foot traveling forward and down in a straight line until the ball contacts the surface (the foot's arch acts as a fulcrum), which creates a launching pad that allows for a solid downstroke with the toes providing traction and balance. The lower leg, the knee, and the thigh, meanwhile, lift and move forward in a straight line powered by muscles in the calf and thigh.

A tape of a dysfunctional foot and leg would show this: As the heel strikes, the foot shears off at an angle instead of falling in a straight line; to keep the walker moving forward, the knee struggles to bring the foot around to where it is supposed to be according to the design of the body, and the result is the weight that would properly fall on the ball of the foot is transmitted somewhere along the inside or outside edges of the foot, which means that our walker is actually performing a skating movement with his feet. At the same time, the lower leg, knee, and thigh are being hoisted off the ground at the hip and swung forward. Aside from the muscles involved in the articulation of the knee joint, all the other gait muscles are taking a free ride at the expense of the hip flexors.

Everted feet are extremely common and it is not necessary for each foot to be everted at the same angle in relationship to the hips. Often one foot points straight ahead while the other goes off at a 15- or 30-degree angle. What's occurring is that one whole side of the body—leg, hip, shoulder—is not engaging. The foot that's straight is on the working, or load-bearing, side of the body. If the heels of your shoes wear unevenly, your feet are everting (or, in rare cases, inverting). This symptom can cause sore and tired feet, poor balance, shin and knee pain, foot cramps and . . . Well, I'll stop there because the list is very long and amounts to just about every foot-related malady. Is it correctable without special shoes or surgery? You bet it is. Stay tuned.

Meanwhile, the thing to remember with the diagnostic process overall is that there are many different ingredients and many different combinations. For starters, though, try to isolate a few key symptoms and ignore the others.

HEADS UP

A third symptom of Condition I which is more difficult to spot without a partner is an out-of-position head. The imaginary grid on your mirror looks like a ladder, but we need to draw in another vertical line that falls exactly halfway between the other two. It runs from the pelvis and goes straight up through the neck to the skull. This line is the spine. It has an S-curve, but at the intersection with the shoulders there is another right angle.

A head that is being pulled forward and down is visible from the side, but as soon as you glance over to the mirror the head changes its position and, therefore, it's difficult to spot. However, you might notice that your chin is down, and if a book was balanced on the top of your head, it would slip off. What's happening is the tilt of the pelvis causes the spine to arch at the low back, one of three spinal "regions" (lumbar, thoracic, cervical). The strong muscles of the groin, the hip flexors, have pulled the pelvis forward and down. Since the spine has the capability of four degrees of flexion built into it, a change at the ground floor, the pelvis, is going to have an impact all along the way, right up to the penthouse: The head comes forward, and gravity starts pulling downward. As the muscles of the neck and upper spine engage to keep the head in place—a job they were not designed to perform—the chin drops because the muscles can't handle the increased load.

Years ago, I starting noticing that the patients I was working with on realigning their heads who were having sinus problems or what they thought of as hay fever attacks would suddenly stop sniffing and snorting to clear their nasal passages. By getting the head back into the functional position, the sinus cavities were level and able to drain. It's logical to assume that the other "systems" of the head, including the basic flow of oxygen to the brain, are similarly impacted.

There is another type of hip (and shoulder) displacement, which is referred to as upper torso rotation (discussed in the next section of this chapter dealing with Condition II, which I recommend you read even if you have already spotted Condition I symptoms). Rotation can occur together with Condition I characteristics, and if it does we must treat that rotation first. If you do detect upper torso rotation (a hip and/or shoulder may appear to be closer to the mirror than its mate), follow the Condition II exercise menu in chapter five (page 127) and then proceed with Condition I after the Condition II symptoms are gone (this should take about a month depending on severity). If you do the recommended Condition II exercises every day for three to four weeks you will be able to see that the rotation is being eliminated; once the mirror shows you that the hip or shoulder is back in place, return to the Condition I routine.

While we are considering a possible mix of symptoms, I should mention that if you see Condition I and III symptoms do the exercise routine for Condition III first, and don't be surprised if a couple of months go by before the symptoms begin to abate. Condition III is a tough customer.

LINKAGE

Throughout a diagnosis, bear in mind that the body is a unit and that it is bifunctional. The forward tilt of the pelvis is a good example. As the shelf of the pelvis angles down in response to the powerful hip flexor muscles, the muscles of the lower back are put under stress. That's where the feeling of tightness comes from in the lower lumbar region. The more you walk with the hip flexors, the more they pull on those lumbar muscles. There is a chain reaction up and down the back. To relieve the tension, there's only one option. We can't deliberately relax our hips, so instead we slump the shoulders and the head. And you've seen it happen (or done it yourself): The tired cowboy wiggles his hips from side to side, raises his shoulders and lets them settle forward while the head nods downward toward the chest.

This maneuver helps take the kinks out of the lower back, but there is a price to be paid. The head and shoulders are forced into a dysfunctional position to accommodate dysfunctional hips and gait-pattern muscles. One dysfunction has given birth to three others. And there's more to come.

The knees and ankles will be prone to stiffness, soreness, and accidental damage. Since the everted foot doesn't function in a forward-back motion it's just hanging out there waiting to snag on something; the "skating" action puts stress on the foot, the ankle, and the knee; if there's a slip or stumble, the flaccid gait muscles aren't strong enough to snap into action and regain the lost balance. In a fall, with the parallel lines and right angles being violated, the knees and ankles are especially vulnerable to injury. The jolt causes lateral stress and torque in addition to the lateral stress and torque already being imposed by the dysfunctional hip.

ABDICATION

At this point, when I'm in my clinic, the question that gets asked most often is "Why do the hip flexors hijack the body?" The answer has two parts. First, the hip flexors are the body's most powerful muscle group. By turning over the walking function to them, you're creating a monster. Those muscles thrive on demand (as do all muscles). But unlike the gait muscles of the leg, which depend on walking to maintain strength and proper function, the hip flexors get a workout even when the body is sitting down by participating in the flexion and extension of the upper body.

Therefore, the muscles of the lower extremities atrophy from disuse while the hip flexors gain strength.

The second part of the answer involves lifestyle. If the way you live and work demands more upper body movement than lower body movement, the gait muscles tend to go. By sitting at a desk all day, the gait muscles are at rest while the hips and upper body continue to move as you type, reach for the phone, or drink a cup of coffee. When you stand up at five o'clock to go home, the hip flexors take over, with the still torpid gait muscles of the leg just hitchhiking along. It doesn't happen suddenly. This abdication by the gait muscles and hip flexor takeover occurs gradually over time.

ON DEMAND

The reason the Egoscue Method is so effective is that it recognizes that functions can be restored by systematically reintroducing demand. Not just any old demand, but demand directed specifically at the dysfunctional muscle groups. The gait muscles, for example, sitting all day under the desk, or standing beside a workbench, are not under demand (or the demand is minimal and inadequate to maintain function). As the hip flexors take over more and more, they start to absorb the marginal demand requirements of walking out to the car or to the cafeteria for lunch. I can't do anything about workplace or lifestyle, but starting in chapter six I will show you how to put demand into the gait muscles and other dysfunctional muscles and joints, no matter how you live or how you work.

Condition II

The map that I'm drawing has only one destination, function, but there are alternate routes. Not everyone needs to visit Condition II. Therefore, it's necessary to go back to the mirror and take another look.

Get comfortable. Let your shoulders and arms settle in. Is one shoulder lower than the other? If not lower, perhaps it seems to be a little closer to the mirror? Does one hand appear to hang lower than the other? When you examine the hands, as they are reflected in the mirror, are you seeing the back of one hand and the thumb of the other?

Also, check your head. We should be able to draw a straight line splitting your forehead, nose and chin, and extending down through your upper torso to the pelvis and floor. It is supposed to divide everything into two exactly equal portions. But if the line angles off at the head or drops down to the left or right of the belly button, it means that the head has been pulled off to one side.

What we're looking for in Condition II is upper torso rotation, which is violating the body's four socket design by allowing the shoulders and hips to swing out of vertical and parallel alignment. The shoulder and hand are the real giveaway characteristics (see figure 17). To see what I mean, roll your shoulders all the way forward into a pronounced slump: Notice how the back of your hands swing around to face forward? In the functional four socket position, the palms of the hands face the sides of the body so that when viewed head-on the thumbs and side of the index fingers are visible. Often, in my clinic, I'll see the thumb and index finger of the patient's left or right hand and all the knuckles and fingers of the other.

As your body reacts to the various environmental factors affecting it, the eyes override the kinesthetic mechanism, which, if functioning properly, would have the head up and the shoulders back. But the eyes are in charge of keeping a level horizon no matter what's going on down below. If it means letting the shoulders and head slump forward—so be it; the kinesthetic sense is of secondary importance to the optical senses.

One scenario that occurs frequently is that the right hip opts out, and when it does, the situation is similar to a ship hitting a rock on the right side; water rushes into the ruptured compartments and the vessel settles into the water listing to the right. Deprived of the right hip, the body also lists to the right; kinesthetically, the head is also being pulled off to the right. But to compensate, to level the horizon, so that we can continue navigating dead ahead, the eyes give the muscles instructions to allow the shoulder to roll forward to adjust the line of travel. It swings around and down, bringing the head with it.

If you're bearing weight on the left side of the body, to name

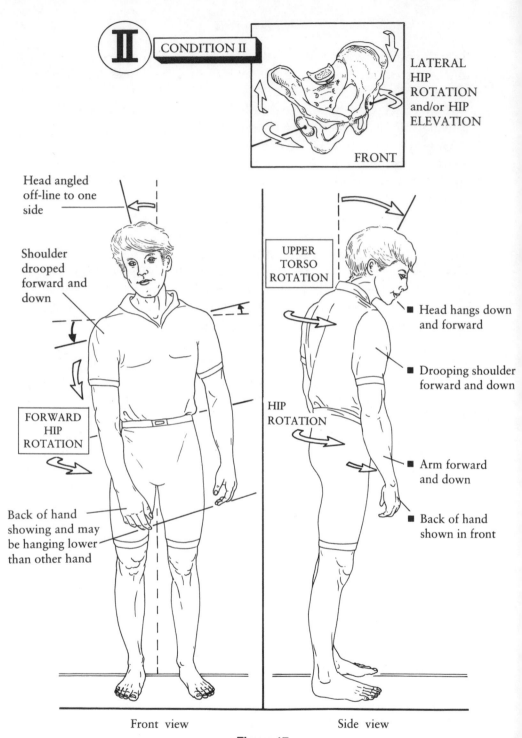

CONDITION II

LATERAL HIP ROTATION and/or HIP ELEVATION

FRONT

Head angled off-line to one side

Shoulder drooped forward and down

UPPER TORSO ROTATION

■ Head hangs down and forward

■ Drooping shoulder forward and down

FORWARD HIP ROTATION

HIP ROTATION

■ Arm forward and down

Back of hand showing and may be hanging lower than other hand

■ Back of hand shown in front

Front view

Side view

Figure 17

another scenario, with the gait muscles of the right side loafing, there is a tendency for the left hip to act as a counterweight and rotate laterally to the right. Think of your trunk in its functional position as the face of a clock with the left hip at 9 and the right hip pointing to 3. The lateral rotation advances the left hip from 9 to 10, and the right hip from 3 to 4. This means that the body wants to fall off to the right when you walk, but our navigational systems are programmed to move us straight ahead. The result is that the upper torso rotates counterclockwise, with the shoulder rolling forward to bring the head and body back into line.

A third scenario to help explain the rotation is a right-handed tennis player who has an inability to bear weight in his right hip. Hence, he doesn't transfer weight in his tennis stroke. To hit the ball, he is always on his front foot. The biomechanics of motion will round the right shoulder forward because the wrong muscles are being used to make the shots. It's being rounded by repetitive misuse.

Whatever the cause, a rotated upper torso looks as though the shoulder is lower and forward of the rest of the body. It's as if you were walking a little sideways, leading with the shoulder (see figure 18). Think of it in terms of a corkscrew that been started into the cork of a wine bottle and twisted a quarter turn, leaving one end of the handle closer to the sommelier.

A quick way to determine whether you have a lateral hip rotation is simply to stand up and immediately look down at your feet before you've had a chance to shift them around. If one foot is ahead of the other, there is rotation. If the left foot is ahead it means that the right hip has slipped out of the 3 o'clock position and moved toward 4. Thus, the right shoulder has probably moved forward and down to compensate.

These symptoms have various manifestations. For one thing, it's not much fun to walk or run. There's a lot of strain on the knees, hips, and shoulders. Often, I see patients who have been told that the cartilage is "gone" from those joints. After I show them photographs of their rotated hips and shoulders, I'll ask, "What if we got rid of that rotation? Maybe you'd stop scouring and scraping away the cartilage if the joint wasn't under such stress." Those photographs are convincing, just as your mirror can be persuasive, and I usually don't have to say much more. Cartilage, I

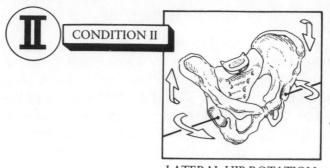

CAUSES:
- HIP OPTS OUT
- BEARING EXTRA WEIGHT ON ONE SIDE OF BODY
- INABILITY TO BEAR WEIGHT ON ONE SIDE

LATERAL HIP ROTATION
and/or HIP ELEVATION

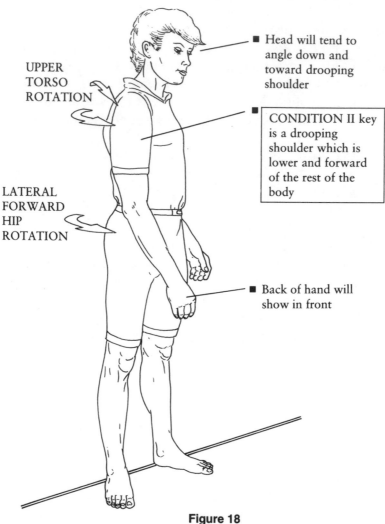

UPPER
TORSO
ROTATION

LATERAL
FORWARD
HIP
ROTATION

- Head will tend to angle down and toward drooping shoulder

- CONDITION II key is a drooping shoulder which is lower and forward of the rest of the body

- Back of hand will show in front

Figure 18
3/4 VIEW

should add, does regenerate in an adult, but only if the individual is functional. Otherwise, he or she just keeps destroying cartilage as fast or faster than it's replaced.

A SOUND INVESTMENT

I want to emphasize that Condition II often piggybacks onto Condition I and/or III. This complicates the diagnosis and treatment process because you might end up thinking that you have to do two different procedures at the same time.

First things first. After suppressing symptomatic pain (see my comments about treating pain in chapter five, pages 82–83), the first step has to be the elimination of the upper torso rotation, otherwise the rotation will counteract the work that's being done on Condition I and II, and maintaining D-lux status. Three or four weeks concentrating on the upper torso rotation should be enough to allow you to move back to the Condition I menu (or III, or D-lux if you are otherwise functional). The timing, however, depends on the severity of the dysfunction. Keep checking the mirror to see whether the rotation is being eliminated. Use your eyes! The dysfunction is clearly visible. Forget the old excuses: "That's just the way God made me."

Don't be in a hurry. It took years to get your body out of its design-shape. A few weeks or months to get it back into functional condition is time well spent.

Condition III

I've saved the worst of the three dysfunctional conditions for last. There was a time when Condition III was relatively unusual. But not any more—and that's a very grim situation indeed.

Take a look at figure 19 to see what I mean. In Condition III, the hips are tilted *under*, which tips the top of the pelvis to the rear as though a pair of hands had gripped the hips from behind, pulling back and down with tremendous force. Imagine the pelvis as a satellite dish with the concave portion pointing straight ahead toward a point on the far horizon. The dysfunction is pulling down and back on the pelvic dish, realigning its concavity upward to the sky at an angle. A principal effect of the hip displacement is to flatten out the S-curve of the spine.

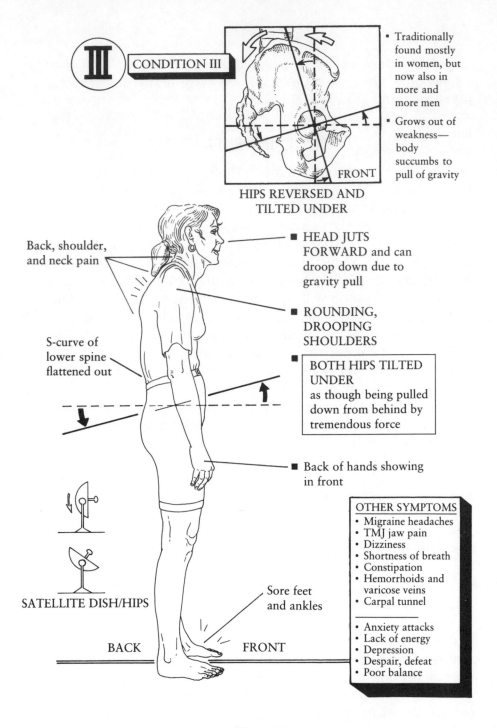

III CONDITION III

- Traditionally found mostly in women, but now also in more and more men
- Grows out of weakness—body succumbs to pull of gravity

FRONT

HIPS REVERSED AND TILTED UNDER

Back, shoulder, and neck pain

■ HEAD JUTS FORWARD and can droop down due to gravity pull

■ ROUNDING, DROOPING SHOULDERS

S-curve of lower spine flattened out

■ BOTH HIPS TILTED UNDER as though being pulled down from behind by tremendous force

■ Back of hands showing in front

OTHER SYMPTOMS
• Migraine headaches
• TMJ jaw pain
• Dizziness
• Shortness of breath
• Constipation
• Hemorrhoids and varicose veins
• Carpal tunnel

• Anxiety attacks
• Lack of energy
• Depression
• Despair, defeat
• Poor balance

SATELLITE DISH/HIPS

Sore feet and ankles

BACK   FRONT

Figure 19
SIDE VIEW

The other characteristics of Condition III are rounded, slumping shoulders and a head that juts forward until it seems like a miracle that the whole body doesn't topple over. You probably recognize what I am describing. It's the posture of despair and dejection, depression and defeat. We see it in photographs of prisoners of war, the homeless, drug addicts, and inmates on death row. But the shocking thing is that I'm finding it more and more on the streets and in shopping malls, the schools and the offices of this country.

To better understand what I'm talking about, try this: Stand up and let your shoulders slump. Bring them forward and down as far as they'll go. Push your hips forward and under by tightening the muscles in your lower back and in the buttocks; the spine will flatten out. Let your head droop down.

How does it feel? Most people say standing that way makes them feel powerless or extremely vulnerable. And that's right on the money. The Condition III person can feel powerless and vulnerable. The body has become so dysfunctional that its structure and systems are literally on the brink of collapse. It's not unusual for the Condition III person to feel lousy—physically and mentally. He or she blames it on old age, bad luck, lack of opportunity, Mom and Dad, the boss, a rotten job, the screaming kids . . . whatever.

Here are some of the symptoms: back, shoulder, and neck pain; poor balance; sore feet and ankles; hemorrhoids and varicose veins; shortness of breath, lack of energy, carpal tunnel, migraine headaches, TMJ pain in the jaw, anxiety attacks, dizziness, constipation, etcetera, etcetera, etcetera.

EQUALITY OF THE SEXES AND GENERATIONS

At one time, it was relatively uncommon to find men with Condition III symptoms. Participation in contact sports and involvement in heavy physical labor, particularly using the upper torso, were seen as male prerogatives. Just recall the almost automatic assumption that men are capable of lifting heavy objects over their heads and that women are not. That bulky carry-on bag gets hoisted into the airplane's overhead rack by the nice man in the aisle seat and he is thanked profusely by the female executive who could run circles around the guy on the jogging track and the office. See what I mean?

Dysfunctions take root whenever we are encouraged and rewarded for restricting our full range of design movement. There is no physiological reason whatsoever to prevent a fully functional woman from heaving that bag into the rack as well as any man.

Let's hear it for chivalry, and let's hear it for women's liberation at the same time. But there's something else at work here. Ironically, the Condition III characteristics that were traditionally associated with "the weaker vessel" are showing up with ever-greater frequency in men. As modern technology alters the environment and reduces the necessity of motion, men are joining women in the Condition III category. Whereas cultural biases once inflicted functional inequality on women, lack of motion has resulted in a perverse form of equality between the sexes—all men and women are becoming equally dysfunctional. Women's liberation arrived too late to save women from dysfunction. "You've come a long way, baby," but you got here after the environment stopped overtly penalizing us for lack of movement. Dysfunction is now a unisex phenomenon. Women shouldn't be surprised if the guy in the aisle seat doesn't volunteer to lift the bag; he may know that the good deed will be rewarded with an aching back or shoulder.

Condition III dysfunctions are also bearing down heavily on our children. Prior to the eighties, Condition III did not exist in high schools, aside from an occasional child suffering from a debilitating congenital illness. Kids were getting enough motion to complete their functional development and carry them through their teen years. Starting sometime in the early to mid-1980s, however, Condition III popped up more frequently, although it was still comparatively unusual. By the late eighties, I had begun to see many instances of it among preteens and teenagers.

HERCULES

Unlike the hip tilt in Condition I, which is caused by strong hip flexor muscles taking over from the gait and posture muscles,

Condition III grows out of weakness. Since many functions have never developed fully or at all, the body's structure and systems are in what amounts to a slow motion free-fall. Gravity is trying to pull everything over and down.

But the body does not give up without a fight. The central nervous system is sending out frantic signals to the few muscles still capable of responding with instructions to do everything possible to keep the body from toppling forward and assuming the fetal position. The pain felt in Condition III, whether in the foot or the jaw or a myriad of other places in between, is a reflection of the herculean effort that is underway. And Hercules himself would have lost the battle against Condition III. No one has jaw muscles or extensor and flexor muscles of the foot capable of preventing a dysfunctional body from folding up like a Swiss army knife.

Take another look at figure 19; the Condition III head is jutting over the toes. There is a muscle in the neck called the playtysma that lowers the lip and tenses the neck. By pulling the head forward and down, the playtysma is stretched tight just because of the position it's in. Now if you tell the playtysma muscle to also help hold the head up, is it any wonder that the Condition III individual has a stiff neck and cramps? What about the permanent frown? If the playtysma's job is to lower the lip, is it surprising that he's forgotten how to smile, or that his lips tremble?

Similarly, the muscles of the foot are designed for bearing weight, keeping the weight balanced, and locomotion. Because we don't use our toes like fingers, there aren't extra opponens muscles in the foot to allow the big and little toes to oppose or to cup the way we cup the palm of the hand. By forcing these specialized muscles to participate in a rescue operation involving the upper torso, Condition III, at the least, is probably going to cause foot cramps, fatigue, and swelling. But that's minor compared to the pain that most Condition III individuals feel in their lower backs, shoulders, and necks.

Condition III has a variety of compensating tricks that can hide dysfunctions. If you look into the mirror and see that your pelvis is thrust forward somewhat, you might be tempted to conclude that your hips are okay. But to keep the body from toppling over, the hips move forward to try to stabilize the center of gravity.

Reach around and feel your low back. If there is no arch or curve, the pelvis is tilted *under* in the classic Condition III position. Fashion models throw their hips forward this way to counteract dysfunctional shoulders and hips—and we've come to think that it looks sexy!

Another way to tell is to stand against a wall or lie on the floor. If the back is instantly flat against the surface, it's a sign of Condition III hip dysfunction.

RESPONSIBILITY

Go back to the mirror. If you see Condition III characteristics, and the side view is particularly revealing, it's time to get busy. Look at your children, spouse, and other family members. As bad as it is, Condition III can be reversed, and there's no difference whether a person is young or old, male or female. More time will be required than with Conditions I and II; not only do we have to restore function, but building strength is also necessary. In advanced cases, Condition III robs an individual of his self-esteem, which makes motivation all that much more difficult. The process, however, once under way, produces abundant positive reinforcement. Just doing something, as opposed to doing nothing, is beneficial. And that is always the first step toward strength and health. It's called taking responsibility.

HARD LABOR FOR PREGNANT WOMEN

I said earlier in this section that Condition III is a unisex phenomenon. However, I want to close with a final comment about women who have this dysfunction. The under-tilt of the hips prevents the pelvis from falling into the natural birthing position, which involves a flaring of the hips forward and down.

Consequently, the baby doesn't drop, and in a biomechanical sense, a pregnant Condition III woman is never ready to give birth, as is her functional sister whose hips swivel around in the final months as she comes to term.

A Condition I woman, I should add, has the opposite problem. Her pelvis is tilted forward by the dysfunction before conception takes place. The body misreads the position as a signal that she is ready to give birth long before the fetus is ready. I tell female Condition I patients that if they intend to have children, they should get the pelvis back into functional position. Otherwise they are risking premature births and miscarriages.

The problem is not premature birth for the Condition III woman, though. Prolonged birth is what's going to happen. Depending on the severity of the hip dysfunction, she is headed for long hours in the delivery room and intense labor pain.

The rising number of caesareans, I believe, is a reflection of the spread of this dysfunction to more and more women. The obstetricians know from the position of the pelvis that there will be trouble and recommend "C-sections"—the physicians assume that nothing can be done about the patient's hips. In my clinic I become a big nag about hips when I'm working with women in their childbearing years because I've found that something can be done. In many cases surgery probably would not be necessary if the hips were repositioned using the Egoscue Method, sparing the mother and child extreme shock and trauma.

D-Lux

On the map that I have been drawing for you, D-lux (figure 20) is the final destination. Ironically, where we want to go most of all is back to our starting place. D-lux is a homecoming. If the energy, exhilaration, and pleasure you feel produce a sense of déjà vu, enjoy it—you *have* been here before, as a child (but your children may not be so lucky).

Make certain that you are, in fact, where you think you are. The mirror doesn't lie. Are the horizontal and vertical lines drawn through your shoulders, hips, knee, and ankles parallel, with right angles at the joints? Is the head centered and the feet straight?

If so, welcome home!

SUBTLE WARNINGS

D-lux amounts to a template with which you can determine whether your body conforms to the design that all human beings inherit from their hunter-gatherer ancestors. It's the points of deviation from the design that lead to dysfunction and pain.

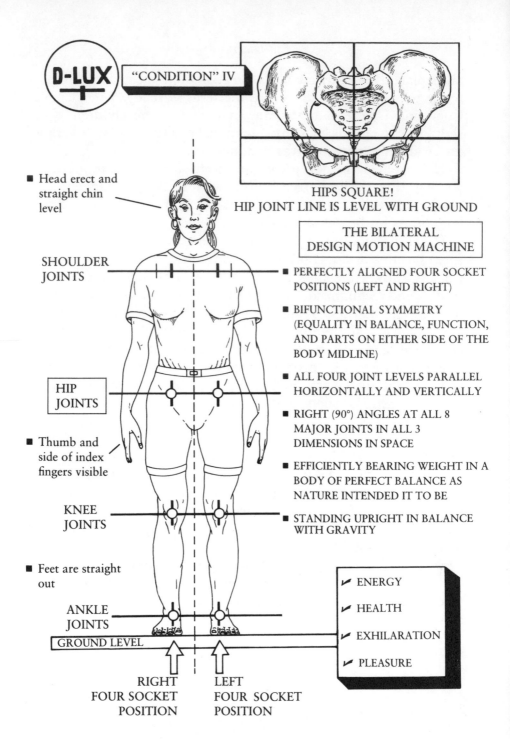

D-LUX "CONDITION" IV

HIPS SQUARE!
HIP JOINT LINE IS LEVEL WITH GROUND

■ Head erect and straight chin level

SHOULDER JOINTS

HIP JOINTS

■ Thumb and side of index fingers visible

KNEE JOINTS

■ Feet are straight out

ANKLE JOINTS

GROUND LEVEL

RIGHT FOUR SOCKET POSITION

LEFT FOUR SOCKET POSITION

THE BILATERAL
DESIGN MOTION MACHINE

■ PERFECTLY ALIGNED FOUR SOCKET POSITIONS (LEFT AND RIGHT)

■ BIFUNCTIONAL SYMMETRY (EQUALITY IN BALANCE, FUNCTION, AND PARTS ON EITHER SIDE OF THE BODY MIDLINE)

■ ALL FOUR JOINT LEVELS PARALLEL HORIZONTALLY AND VERTICALLY

■ RIGHT (90°) ANGLES AT ALL 8 MAJOR JOINTS IN ALL 3 DIMENSIONS IN SPACE

■ EFFICIENTLY BEARING WEIGHT IN A BODY OF PERFECT BALANCE AS NATURE INTENDED IT TO BE

■ STANDING UPRIGHT IN BALANCE WITH GRAVITY

✔ ENERGY

✔ HEALTH

✔ EXHILARATION

✔ PLEASURE

Figure 20
THE FUNCTIONAL DESIGN POSTURE

In chapter five you will find a series of exercises which will allow you to maintain your D-lux membership.

Why bother if your body is functional and in proper alignment? I know how tempting it is to let things slide. If it ain't broke why fix it? But changes in our environment and lifestyle take place gradually and often go unnoticed. Another old cliché, "an ounce of prevention is worth a pound of cure," has a lot of truth to it.

Unfortunately, we're not pinball machines with a buzzer and a sign that flashes "Tilt!" whenever the mechanism is being abused. Our warnings, initially, are more subtle. But we've been taught how to ignore them with things like aspirin and knee braces. Other louder messages have been superimposed: "Of course you're stiff after riding in an airplane seat for three hours . . ." or, "My ankles swell up pretty bad when I fly because of the altitude." In both cases, overall lack of movement is to blame, not the cramped seat or the altitude (dehydration is also a prime factor in the swelling, as it is in jet lag), but we can't hear the body tell us that because of all the noise. Finally, to get our attention, it shouts at us in the form of acute pain; then we panic and run to someone who promises to make the pain go away.

D-lux, whether it has been achieved through the Egoscue Method or by way of an environment that still requires enough movement to maintain the body's design functions, turns up the volume. We can hear what the body is saying to us over all the distracting noise, and if a time comes when there's pain, even though the D-lux template checks out, it's obvious that important information is being communicated, information that must not be ignored. Furthermore, the increased volume may even be telling you that it's time to see a physician. The body knows when it's sick and in trouble.

5

Restoring and Maintaining Function and Flexibility

I have already broken out the Condition I, II, III, and D-lux characteristics. Now let's run through a few more procedural fine points and then move on to the exercise "menu" for each.

In a normal week at my clinic I draw on literally hundreds of different exercises. I have made some of them up from scratch, others are borrowed from yoga or are updated versions of moves going back to elementary school physical education classes, and there are variations on familiar workout routines.

If I tried to reproduce every one of them here, I'd be falling into the trap that I decried at the beginning of the book: Complexity would take over. We'd be smothered by it. In the clinic, I have the luxury of fine-tuning the treatment routine. I can see how each patient reacts and adjust the program accordingly. If the circumstances warrant, I can improvise to get an injured professional athlete back on the duty roster as quickly as possible. A book, however, requires a more conservative approach.

Even so, the Egoscue Method works despite the fact that I've never met you. It works because of the four categories that I have identified. Think of that for a moment—four conditions. Not four hundred or four million. And *every* person fits into one of those categories. The diagnostic and treatment process, therefore, stops being an incredibly cumbersome pursuit of ever more elusive symptoms.

Thanks to the four categories, the exercises described below get the job done with a minimum of fuss. And you will notice that none of them are all that demanding physically. This is not a body-building program. But some of the moves will be more difficult than others. A lot depends on your individual dysfunctions. The exercises that are toughest are telling you about the severity of the dysfunction. Very often, as well, an exercise will be harder on one side of the body than it is on the other. Again, that's valuable information about what's going on in your back, hips, shoulders, or wherever.

A workout lasting about an hour each day should be sufficient. It won't be long before you begin seeing and feeling results. Jane, who came out to the clinic last year from Washington, D.C., with a hip and shoulder rotation, had her rounded shoulders flat on the floor after two sessions with her exercise menu.

THE WEIGHT TEST

Now, what happens if nothing happens? Suppose you do the exercises and there seems to be no improvement. What then? If that's the case, and there really is no improvement, you may be living proof that the Egoscue Method cannot be taught through a book. However, I don't believe that to be the case, otherwise I wouldn't have spent hundreds of hours writing this one.

My advice is to step back and assess the situation. Ask yourself, "Am I being too impatient?" One way to test for impatience is to do a before-and-after check of your weight distribution. Stand on a hard surface in bare feet; close your eyes, breathe from the diaphragm, and relax. Where is the weight in your feet? Where do you feel it: the heels, the inside edge, the outside edge, or the balls of the feet? Identify where the weight is in both feet. If you're functional, D-lux, you will immediately know that the weight in both feet is on the balls of the feet. If you are dysfunctional it will be somewhere else, and probably it will be different for each foot.

Okay, do your exercises, and at the end repeat the weight test. If the weight distribution is different, if it's shifting toward the functional position, you are making progress. The exercises are working. Stick with it.

No change? What I think is going on in that case is that your dysfunctions aren't ready for treatment. You may not be feeling pain, and that's deceptive. If you were in pain, we wouldn't be doing anything other than three basic exercises to suppress it (static back press, the supine groin, and the air bench, which will be described later in this chapter, following a detailed discussion of pain). We have to get rid of the pain before treatment can begin and that's what those exercises do. However, without pain it seems as if the dysfunctions are under control enough to allow for the next step. That may not be true, if you don't think there is progress.

If you have doubts go back and reread the diagnostic chapter. You may have misdiagnosed the dysfunctions. Perhaps you have overlooked Condition II upper torso rotation. Have a friend or family member take a look; a second opinion is always helpful. Above all, trust your instincts. The body will tell you what's going on. Those four sets of characteristics amount to a language, a simple, eloquent language that is within our power to understand.

BLAMESMANSHIP

These exercises can't do it alone. You need to take responsibility for your health. If you are unable to find the time to do the routine, don't blame the exercises. If you take short cuts and only work on one side of the body, don't blame the exercises. If you disregard the prescribed sequence, don't blame the exercises.

Is there a glaring contradiction here? How can you take the responsibility when I make demands like this?

To answer that question, let me focus on the sequence of the exercises as an example. By studying the musculoskeletal system for more than two decades, I've learned the limitations of doing blanket, generic exercises that presume to treat equally all the major and minor muscle groups in one part of the body. If the body was functional, there'd be no problem: The right muscles would move the bones to the right places. But once dysfunction sets in that doesn't happen any longer. The prescribed sequence is isolating specific muscle groups and telling them to get busy or to butt out. If a function is performed by, let's say three muscle groups, the message has got to go to all three in the proper order, otherwise it will be garbled.

If you say, "No, Pete, I'm taking responsibility now. From my exercise menu, I'm only going to do the static back press, the runner's stretch, and the downward dog. Those three make me feel better," my response is: Go ahead. They probably do make you feel better. The pain symptoms are being suppressed; even so, the problem remains. Ask yourself why you aren't doing the others, and doing them in the correct order. Could it be that the others aren't providing you with as quick a fix? Is it too much trouble to do the full sequence?

In my clinic I'm always on watch for signs that the patient is trying to transfer responsibility to me or to the exercises. And since this book is a surrogate for my clinic, I am particularly concerned that you don't get the mistaken impression that the Egoscue Method is going to fix your back or knee or shoulder.

No way. *You're* going to do the fixing.

YOUR ITINERARY

Earlier, I used the analogy of a road map. Let's stay with it as I outline the exercises by using a destination and a route for each exercise. The destination is what we are setting out to achieve; the specific instructions on how to get there make up the route. The exercises are arranged alphabetically. I've tagged each one to identify the condition which it applies to and where it falls in the menu sequence (e.g., Condition II, exercise 4). Jot down the menu on a separate sheet of paper, and use small self-stick removable notes to mark the pages describing the exercises on your menu. In a few days you'll know the sequence and the routines by heart and won't have to refer to the book for instructions.

If you have a mish-mash of symptoms, "all of the above–none of the above," don't despair. Many people have various combinations of symptoms. Condition I is the most common category. But as I said in the previous chapter, if there are Condition II symptoms present go after them first. The muscles of a Condition II person tend to be tight; the exercises will loosen things up and provide the flexibility for the Condition I or III remediation routines.

Once you've identified and treated Condition II characteristics, then look for Condition III symptoms. If you spot them, consider yourself to be Condition III and follow the appropriate menu. Once those symptoms are gone, move to the Condition I routine.

I want to warn you away from window shopping through the

other sequences or the whole list of exercises. If an exercise is not on your menu, it's because I've found that the exercise does not address your dysfunctions. And I am definitely posting the no trespassing sign on D-lux. If you are in Conditions I, II, or III and climb the fence into D-lux territory before you're functional— trespassers will be prosecuted with *pain,* and it will be your body acting as judge and jury.

MORE ABOUT PAIN

The time has come to specifically address the pain symptom in regard to diagnosis and the restoration of function.

If you are feeling pain in an ankle, knee, hip, shoulder, or back, that symptom *must* be tackled first no matter what the diagnosed condition. Diagnostically, the pain is helpful in that it provides confirmation that there is a problem. However, don't be tricked into believing that the problem can be resolved at the site of the pain. In terms of treatment, we have to put out the fire and then change the fuses that led to the short circuit and the conflagration.

For those who are hurting somewhere (musculoskeletal pain), start with the static back press, supine groin stretch, and air bench *until the pain ceases,* and then begin at the top of the appropriate sequence, but try not to push the number of repetitions to the threshold of pain—you'll feel it coming on if you pay attention to what the body is saying. Should the pain return, don't ignore it. Interrupt the routine and use those exercises I just named to suppress it. For a while you may only be able to do those three, but that's okay. Every minute you spend with your hips and shoulders back in the proper position is much like accumulating "frequent flyer" mileage. One day it all adds up: You get to upgrade and move on without pain.

These three exercises can also be added to the end of the full sequence for a comfortable way to wind up the routine.

If there was so much pain that you had trouble standing in front of the mirror to do a self-diagnosis, go immediately to the three pain-suppression exercises and save the self-diagnosis for later. The static back press, in particular, will give you relief if you give it enough time to work.

That is an extremely important point about pain: Unless you take responsibility, the pain and the dysfunction will continue.

The exercises can't do it without you. I'd hate to hear, "Well, I got down in the static back press for five minutes and my back still hurt." The hip and back have got to be given enough time to settle down to become flat on the floor. Gravity will do it, but sometimes, depending on the severity of the dysfunction, it can take two hours or more. Is it worth two hours? I can't answer that question. Only you can. Unfortunately, there are people who'd say, "No, hand me the Valium." The decision has to be made by each person. But I can tell you, based on my experience, once function begins to return, it will get faster and easier to suppress the pain. Two hours today may be ninety minutes tomorrow. After a few weeks, it could be fifteen minutes. Perhaps there will be setbacks; even so, the line of travel will be headed for function and fitness—if that is where you are determined to go.

D & D

Before I present the Egoscue Method exercises, I'll give you an important list of do's and don'ts:

- **Do** remember the four socket position; shoulders, hips, knees, and ankles should be in line, feet pointed straight ahead; the head should also be back.
- **Don't** forget to breathe with your diaphragm and use your stomach; not shallow little puffs, make your lungs fill the chest cavity.
- **Do** take off your shoes, except where I have indicated otherwise; give the muscles of the foot a workout.
- **Don't** forget that the body is a bilateral machine; an exercise that's done on one side of the body *must* be done on the other. No short cuts.
- **Do** engage and activate your muscles. Make them talk to you.
- **Don't** provoke or ignore intense nerve or muscle pain.
- **Do** *the exercises in sequence* since each one prepares the body for the next. No picking and choosing.

By reading this far you've had your ticket punched; so let's go on the most important journey you'll ever take.

Abdominals (Wall Crunchies)
Condition I, exercise 5
Condition II, exercise 8
D-lux, exercise 6

Destination: Wall crunchies energize the abdominal muscles, but a full traditional situp doesn't do that because the powerful hip flexors kick in after about six degrees of elevation. Hence, the situp crazies at the gym are building terrific hip flexors when what they're really trying to do is flatten their stomachs. You may have noticed that after a long series of traditional situps, you'll start coming off the mat or bench sideways, with either the right or left shoulder leading. That's the hip flexors showing their strength, and it indicates which side of the body is doing most of the load bearing work. We've got to curb the excesses of the hip flexors and convince the abdominals to help out with the flexion and extension of the low back.

Route: (Start with 1 set of 25 and build to 2 sets of 50.) Lie on your back with both feet on a wall, knees at a 90 degree angle. The feet should be in line with the knees, and knees in line with the hips (figure 21). Clasp your hands behind the base of the head. Let the head relax in the hands while looking at the ceiling. Lift the shoulders and head off the floor while exhaling. Lift as high as you can using only the abdominals, not the hip flexors. Keep your lower back flat throughout the motion.

If you notice the hips or knees moving up and down, the feet coming off the wall a bit or that you're really pushing hard on the wall with your feet, then you're using the hip flexors rather than the abdominals. Make sure you don't yank on the neck, and that the shoulders lift off the floor.

Another way to insure that the hip flexors are neutralized is to concentrate on keeping eye contact with the ceiling. When the eye contact is broken, it means that your head and upper back are off the floor to the point that the abdominals have handed off the lifting motion to the hip flexors.

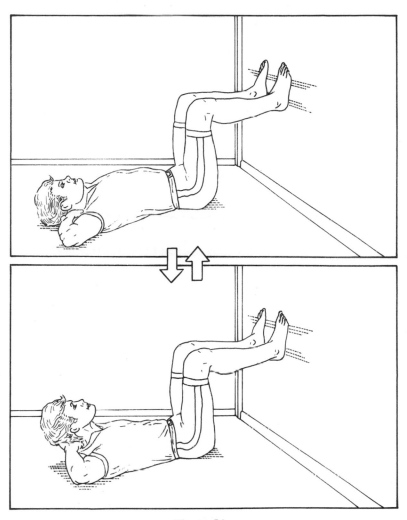

Figure 21
ABDOMINALS

Air Bench
CONDITION I, EXERCISE 10
CONDITION II, EXERCISE 13
D-LUX, EXERCISE 19

Destination: We want the muscles of your thighs to get the idea that they are supposed to be supporting the trunk. If you have trouble with this one initially, welcome to the club! A lot of people have difficulty because it forces their leg muscles, instead of the hip flexors, to do the work of holding the body off the ground. Skiers like the air bench because they discover that turning becomes a lot easier when the thigh muscles take part.

Route: (Hold 1 to 3 minutes.) Stand against a wall with the small of the back and the hips pressing the wall. Place your feet a shoulder-width apart in front of the wall. Make sure the feet are far enough away from the wall so that when you bend your knees they are above the ankles, not the toes. Bend the knees and lower the body down the wall (figure 22). Push against the wall with your lower back to feel the quadriceps working (the strain should be felt equally in both the right and left thighs). If you have pain in the kneecaps, slide up the wall a bit. Do not bend the knees to less than a 90-degree angle. Check to make sure that your feet stay straight and the knees are in line with the feet, rather than flaring in or out.

Breathe! To come out of this, use your hands to push off the wall, and then walk around for a minute.

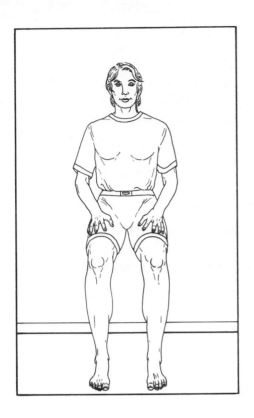

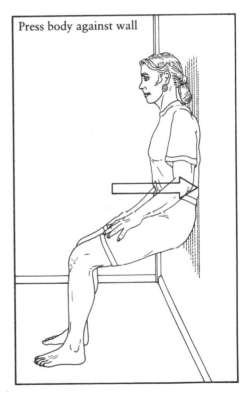

Press body against wall

Figure 22
AIR BENCH

Arm Circles
CONDITION I, EXERCISE 1
CONDITION II, EXERCISE 1
CONDITION III, EXERCISE 1
D-LUX, EXERCISE 1

Destination: The arm circles are strengthening the muscles of the upper back, the ones involved in the ball and socket work of the shoulder, to give them the ability to compete in the tug of war with your hip flexors. This is such an "easy" exercise that you might be tempted to skip it to save time. But your shoulders won't break out of their forward slump if the ball and socket function isn't energized. And it won't be easy for many people with severe shoulder dysfunctions.

Route: (Start with 25 and build to 75 in each direction.) Stand erect with your head up, feet squared, and arms at sides. Your hands are in the golfer's grip, that is, fingers curled in, knuckles flexed and thumbs extended.

Raise the arms out to the side making sure both shoulders remain even (figure 23). As long as both shoulders are even, lift your arms up to shoulder level, parallel to the floor. If a shoulder "pops up" or rolls forward, lower the arms back to the level where both shoulders are even.

In this position, squeeze your shoulder blades together slightly. With palms facing down toward the floor (thumbs pointed forward), rotate the arms in an approximately six inch diameter circle forward, toward the extended thumbs. To reverse the circles, turn your palms to face the ceiling and circle backward, toward the extended thumbs.

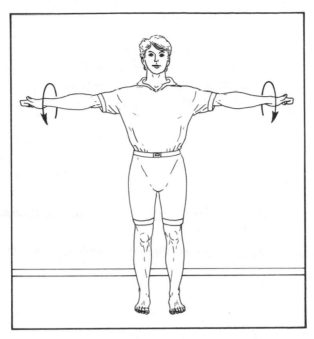

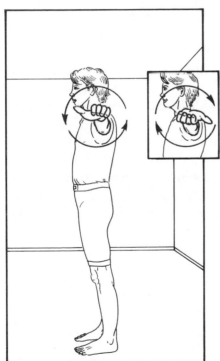

LOWER ARMS IF SHOULDER "POPS"
OR ROLLS FORWARD AT
SHOULDER LEVEL

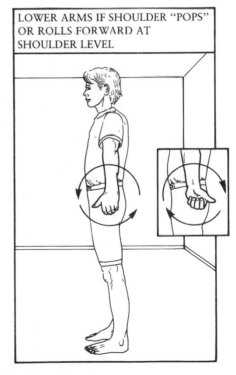

Figure 23
ARM CIRCLES

Cats and Dogs
CONDITION I, EXERCISE 7
CONDITION III, EXERCISE 2
D-LUX, EXERCISE 3, 5, 15

Destination: We need to convince your shoulders and hips that they can work together again. You may feel a little silly doing this one, but it's even sillier not to do the exercise. Cats and Dogs feels good, because the exercise is activating all the posture muscles of the back from the shoulders down to the hips. There is a wonderful ripple effect from top to bottom and bottom to top, just like a pianist running his fingers up and down the keyboard of a piano. The hips and shoulders are participating in the flexion and extension of the spine.

Route: (1 set of 15.) Get on your hands and knees into a position that forms a right angle box (figure 24). The hands should be directly under the shoulders and knees under the hips (make sure the knees are spread far enough apart to line up with the hips). Your weight should be evenly distributed and feet relaxed.

    Smoothly round up the back and curl the head under—like a cat with an arched back; then smoothly sway the back down as the head looks up—like a contented dog. Make one continuous movement, rather than holding in each spot. Keep your arms straight. Exhale as the head curls under and inhale as the head looks up.

    Your shoulders and hips are working together in this exercise. In series it looks like a line of speed bumps alternating with potholes: upward arch–downward sway–upward arch–downward sway. In the dog portion there is more involved than just bringing the head up and allowing the back to flatten. The hips and shoulders should be pressing the back down into a slight trough.

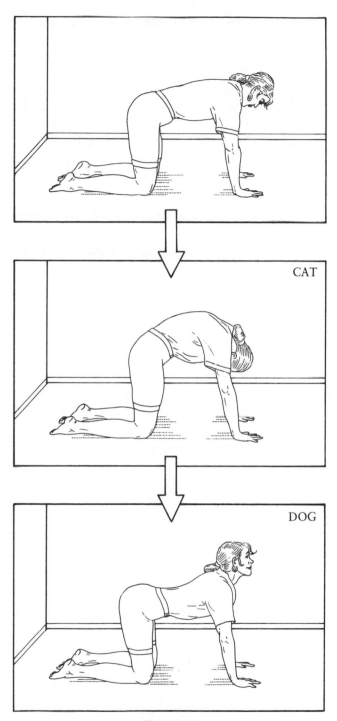

CAT

DOG

Figure 24
CATS AND DOGS

Crocodile Twist
CONDITION II, EXERCISE 10

Destination: We are going to be promoting bilateral activity by literally wringing out the posture muscles of the spine and the hip, making them contract and release equally on both sides—something they've forgotten how to do because of upper torso rotation. Listen to your body on this one (and all the others as well). If it starts to hurt take the crocodile twist out of the sequence and substitute a static back exercise. After a couple of days try the twist again, but go easy.

Route: (Hold 30 seconds to 1 minute each side.) Lie on your back with legs extended. Put your right foot on top of the toes of your left foot (the heel should ride on the tip of the big toe). Extend your arms out to the sides level with shoulders, palms facing into the floor (figure 25).

Tighten the quadriceps of both legs and roll your feet to the left, trying to get them to touch the floor, while keeping one foot on top of the other. As you do this, lift your right hip off the floor, trying to get it to point to the ceiling. Your head looks to the right. Hold this position and breathe; keep the quadriceps tight. Reverse the feet and repeat on the other side.

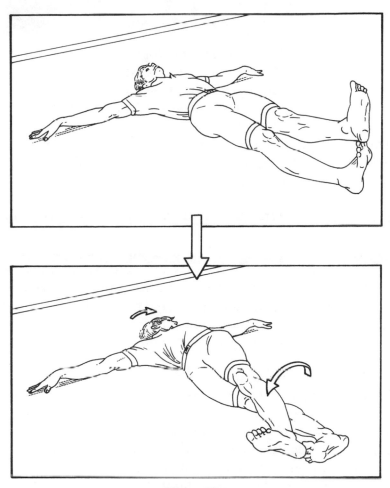

Figure 25
CROCODILE TWIST

Downward Dog
CONDITION I, EXERCISE 8
CONDITION II, EXERCISE 3
D-LUX, EXERCISE 7

Destination: We're giving the posterior muscles from head to foot a wake-up call. All those muscle groups are being forced to engage, instead of allowing a few of the more powerful muscles to have all the fun. After a long drive, a day behind the desk, or an airplane ride this exercise is terrific for getting the kinks out.

Route: (Hold for 30 seconds to 1 minute.) Begin in the same hands and knees position as for Cats and Dogs; your hands should be directly under the shoulders and knees spread apart directly under the hips. Curl your toes under and raise the torso up so that you are now off your knees and on your hands and feet. The configuration will be a triangle, with your hips at the apex (figure 26).

Make sure that the hands do not move back toward the feet. Push the hips back and tighten the quadriceps as you gently lower the heels to the floor. You should feel this stretch in your calves. Check to make sure your feet are parallel, shoulder-width apart, that the quadriceps are tight, and that the hips are pushing up and back over the heels. The back must be flat, not bowed. Breathe! If you cannot lower the heels to the floor, do what you can while still keeping the legs tight; it may take a couple of weeks but they will eventually come down to the floor. There should be no pain in the back or hips.

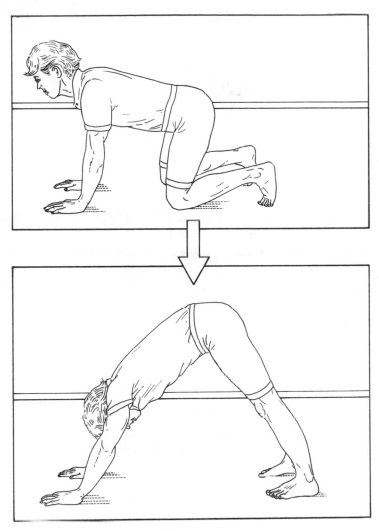

Figure 26
DOWNWARD DOG

Elbow Curls
CONDITION I, EXERCISE 2
D-LUX, EXERCISE 2

Destination: Elbow curls are a way to rejuvenate the muscles of the upper back and remind the shoulder that it has a hinge function as well as a ball and socket. Furthermore, we're telling the hinge that it moves forward and back.

Route: (Start with 10 and build to 20.) Using both hands and the golfer's grip (fingers curled inward at the second knuckle joint, thumbs extended as though you were about to hitch a ride), place the flat ridges formed by the area between the first and second knuckle joints along your temples with thumbs extended down the cheeks. Check to make sure your feet are square and then bring your elbows together to touch in front (figure 27). Take the elbows back level with your shoulders. We should be able to draw a straight line from your left elbow across the top of your shoulders to the right elbow. The head should remain still and your knuckles remain on your temples. If this motion is difficult to do without head movement—it may rock back and forth—stand with your back against a wall with your head touching the surface at all times as the elbows come together and then return to the wall. Keep your shoulder blades against the wall.

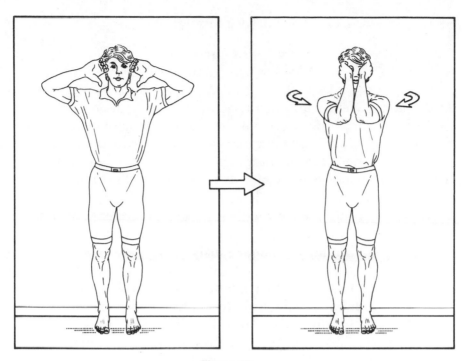

Figure 27
ELBOW CURLS

Extended Lateral
D-LUX, EXERCISE 9

Destination: We're engaging the gait pattern muscles on one side of the body and, at the same time, we're stretching the muscles of the other hip. This is a D-lux exercise. The body is designed for unilateral hip activity. The best example is one that we probably have all encountered: It's a nice day for a walk. I'm climbing up a mountain path and come to a fallen tree trunk. I put my left foot up on the tree and push off with my right to scramble over the obstacle. Each hip is doing something different—one stretching, the other load bearing—simultaneously.

Route: (Hold 45 seconds to 1 minute.) Stand in the triangle position with your back to the wall, feet spread wider than the hips, and both feet straight ahead. Turn the left foot out to the side so that it is perpendicular to the straight foot (see the triangle exercise below for more). With the left foot turned out, bend the knee, making sure the knee goes out directly over the toes rather than rolling inward. Place your left hand flat on the floor beside and outside the left foot. The right leg remains straight and the quadriceps are tight. Extend the right arm over the right ear and face the palm toward the floor (figure 28). Do not allow the right hip to roll forward and away from the wall. Once in this position, check to make sure the right leg is contracted, the hip is not turned forward, the left hand is on the floor beside the left foot, and the right arm is stretching over the right ear with the palm facing down toward the floor.

Breathe! To release this stretch, turn the right hip toward the floor as you bring your right arm to the floor and bend your right knee to touch the floor. Stand up and reverse the directions on the other side.

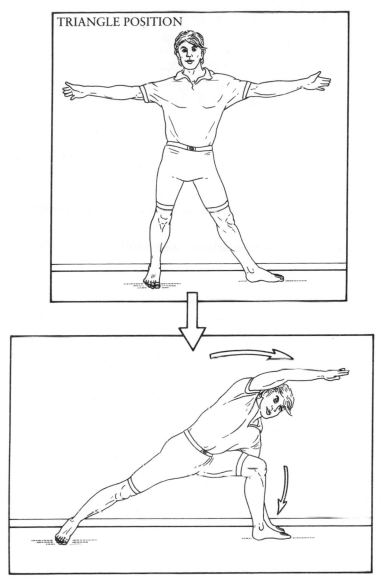

Figure 28
EXTENDED LATERAL

Foot Circles and Point Flexes
CONDITION I, EXERCISE 6
CONDITION II, EXERCISE 9
CONDITION III, EXERCISE 5
D-LUX, EXERCISE 11

Destination: These exercises are waking up the muscles of the foot, ankle, and lower leg so that they can start operating in the proper gait pattern—proper for humans rather than proper for waterfowl. With eversion, your feet aren't flexing properly; they're rolling inward from the ankle joint. You'll probably be surprised at how much work this is going to be. But it also feels good to have this function restored.

Route: (20 circles, each way, and build to 40; 10 point/flex, and build to 20.) Lie on your back with your left leg extended and your right leg bent toward the chest. Clasp your hands behind the bent knee and draw it toward your chest until the lower leg is parallel to the floor. Support the knee in that position while you circle the right foot the designated number of times. Reverse and circle the other way (figure 29).

Make sure the knee stays absolutely still so that the circular movement is at the ankle, not the knee.

For point and flex, bring the toes back toward the shin to flex the foot, and then reverse the direction to point your foot. Again, the knee doesn't move. When the foot circles and point/flexes are completed on one foot, change to the other foot.

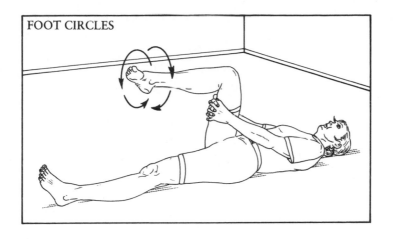

FOOT CIRCLES

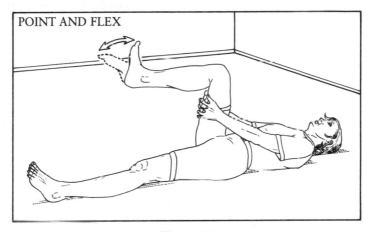

POINT AND FLEX

Figure 29
FOOT CIRCLES AND POINT FLEXES

Frog
CONDITION II, EXERCISE 5
D-LUX, EXERCISE 20

Destination: This is a pelvic exercise, working on the groin and adductor muscles on the inside of the leg. In Condition III, those muscles are weak individually and they interact poorly, if at all. We're strengthening them and reintroducing design-function movement.

Route: (Hold 1 to 2 minutes.) Lie on your back, pull your feet toward your torso and put the soles of your feet together, letting the knees turn out. Make sure the feet are centered in the middle of the body (figure 30). The lower back does not have to be flat into the floor, but you should not feel pain in the back. Relax the legs and feel a stretch in the inner thighs and groin.

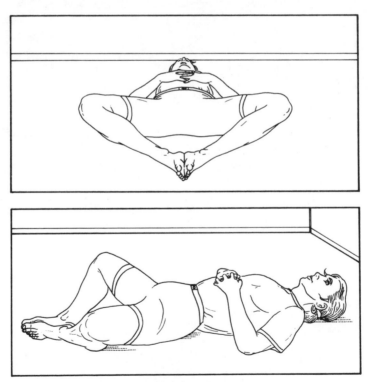

Figure 30
FROG

Gravity Drop *(with scapular contractions)*
CONDITION II, EXERCISE 2

Destination: This is my clinic's secret weapon for dealing with lateral hip rotation. It repositions the hip, encourages the muscles of the upper back to rescue the head from falling forward, and tells the shoulders that it's not necessary to rotate laterally in order to keep the body moving in a straight line.

Route: (3 sets of 20 contractions.) You'll need to go to a staircase for this one, and put on rubber soled shoes for traction. Stand on the stairs as though you were climbing upward. Your feet should be parallel, a shoulder-width apart. Hold onto the rail with one

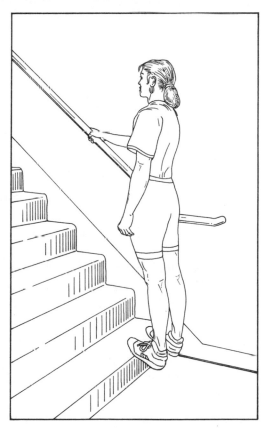

Figure 31
GRAVITY DROP

hand and edge backward until your heels are off the stair tread and hanging in midair (figure 31). Keep easing back so that your weight falls on the balls of your feet. More than half of each foot should be off the tread. Hang on! This is not a balance exercise.

Check your feet again. They should be parallel, straight ahead and a shoulder-width apart. Put downward pressure on the heels to engage the posterior muscles of the leg. You should feel them tighten, and they will drop lower than the leading edge of the stair tread—but don't force down hard on the heels. Bring your shoulders back and level. Bend the free arm at the elbow to 90 degrees and raise it so that the back of your hand is near your chin. With this arm and the one that's holding the rail (let the hand slide back and forth a little), slowly squeeze the shoulder blades together and release. Don't be in a hurry or use a jerky, snapping motion on the shoulder blades.

Hip Crossover
D-LUX, EXERCISE 17

Destination: Hips are hips, but they're not equally hip. One (or both) of them, when there is lateral rotation, is in the wrong place. This is a D-lux exercise, so rotation isn't a problem, and we're out to keep it that way.

Route: (Hold 30 seconds to 1 minute.) Lie on your back with both knees bent and feet flat on the floor. Cross the right ankle over the left knee and press the right knee out toward the feet (figure 32). While maintaining this position, lower your right foot to the left side and place it flat on the floor. The left knee stays bent and both feet flat on the floor. Keep the right knee pressing up towards the ceiling to feel a stretch in the area of your right hip. Come out of this the same way you went into it. Reverse the directions and repeat on the other side.

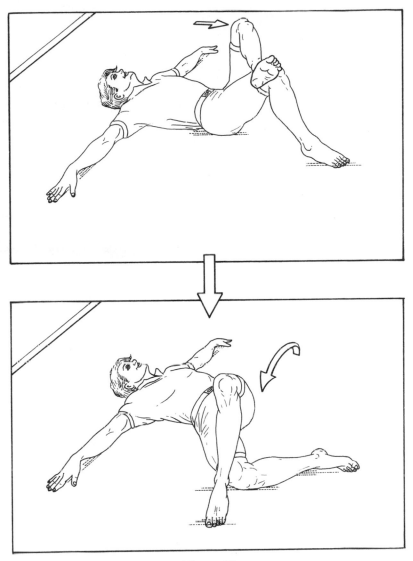

Figure 32
HIP CROSSOVER

Hip Lift
D-lux, exercise 18

Destination: Without being too technical, what's happened with the dysfunction addressed by this exercise is that there is a limited-motion joint, a component of the hip, that has flared out in such a way as to force the femur to rotate to the inside, dragging the knee along with it. The knee is pointing inward instead of straight ahead. The hip lift counteracts the out-flaring of the joint.

Route: (Hold 30 seconds to 1 minute.) Lie on your back with both knees bent and feet flat on the floor. Cross the right ankle over the left knee and press the right knee out toward the feet.

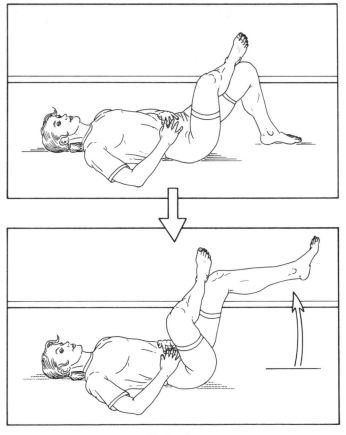

Figure 33
HIP LIFT

While maintaining this position, lift the left leg toward the chest (figure 33). Make sure your hips stay on the floor. Hold this position as you breathe. Check to insure that the right knee is still pressing out and the left knee is in line with the left shoulder, with your hips still on the floor. You should feel a stretch in the right hip. Reverse the directions and repeat on the other side.

Isolated Hip Flexor Lifts
D-LUX, EXERCISE 4

Destination: You may be right handed or left handed, but not right hipped or left hipped. We need to get both of them doing the

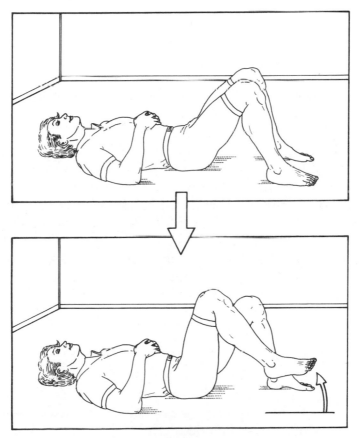

Figure 34
ISOLATED HIP FLEXOR LIFTS

same amount of work and moving outward from the medial plane of the body in a straight line.

Route: (Start with 3 sets of 5; build to 3 sets of 20.) Lie on your back with the knees bent and your feet flat on the floor. Ready? Lift one foot 6 to 8 inches off the floor. Keep the knee in line with the shoulder and the foot in line with the knee (figure 34). Perform the designated number of repetitions in one set, and then repeat with the other leg. Keep alternating sets between each leg until the designated amount of sets is completed. Make sure you don't lift the knee too high. You should feel the hip flexors doing the work rather than the abdominals or quadriceps.

Pelvic Tilts
CONDITION II, EXERCISE 11

Destination: The muscles of the lower back are being asked to go to work, instead of subordinating themselves to the hips and the muscles of the two other spinal regions.

Route: (1 set of 10.) Lie on your back with knees bent, feet flat on the floor and hands resting at your sides. Roll your hips toward your head to flatten your lower back into the floor. Do not lift your hips off the floor. Then roll your hips away to make the lower back arch off the floor, creating a space between the floor and your back (figure 35).

Do these rolls in a smooth continuous motion, flattening the back into the floor and rolling the lower back off the floor. Remember to breathe as you move the hips forward and back.

Push-Ups
D-LUX, EXERCISE 10

Destination: You know where we're going with this one—Parris Island. Seriously, a push-up doesn't only involve arms and shoulders. All the muscles from hip to shoulder have got to join in the effort, otherwise a sway back develops, which indicates that the muscles along the spine and elsewhere aren't taking part.

Route: (Start with 5 and build to 30.) Lie on your stomach with the elbows bent. Put your hands palm down on the floor, approximately 6 inches wider than the shoulders and in a straight line with the shoulders. Hands should be parallel to the body with fingers toward the head. Curl your toes under and straighten your arms to raise the entire body up as one straight unit. Bend the elbows to lower the body toward the floor. Keep the head in line with the spine. Exhale as you straighten the arms. It is important to remember to keep the entire length of the body absolutely straight. Do a comfortable amount of repetitions. This means as many as you can do without losing the correct form. As you become stronger, gradually increase the repetitions weekly.

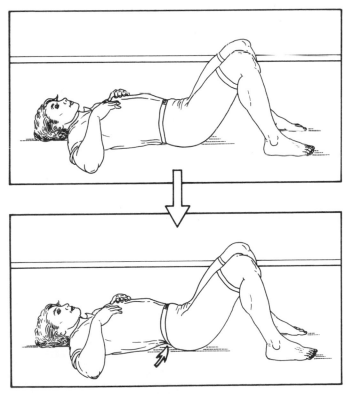

Figure 35
PELVIC TILTS

Quadratus Lumborum Stretch (QLO)
D-LUX, EXERCISE 12

Destination: What we're setting out to do here is to put lateral motion in the spine from a stable pelvic position.

Route: (Hold 30 seconds to 1 minute each side.) Sit on the floor with your legs straight and spread apart. Make sure you are sitting

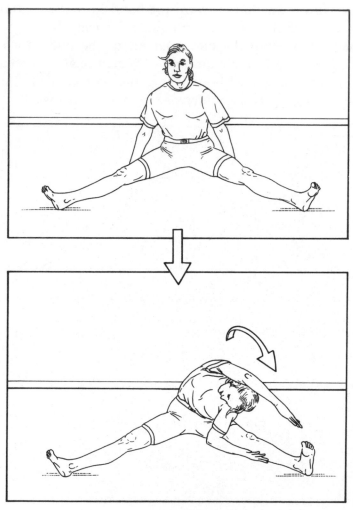

Figure 36
QUADRATUS LUMBORUM STRETCH

straight up over the hips and not rolling backward. Flex your feet so that the feet and knees are pointing straight up. Bend your left elbow and place it along the inside of your left leg near the knee with the palm facing up. Slide it under the left calf. Extend your right arm over your right ear, bending sideways over your left leg, and twisting your upper torso slightly. Try to touch your toes with your right arm (figure 36). Hold and breathe as you check to make sure the knees and toes are pointing to the ceiling and the quadriceps are contracted. Reverse the directions and repeat on the other side.

Runner's Stretch
CONDITION I, EXERCISE 9 (MODIFIED)
CONDITION II, EXERCISE 4 (MODIFIED)
D-LUX, EXERCISE 13 (REGULAR)

Destination: This is an old standby. Many people use it to warm up before running and then to cool down. It's designed to isolate the hamstrings and let them know how long they are so they can perform their walking and running movements in coordination with the hip. Squeeze the quads equally.

Route: (Hold 30 seconds to 1 minute.) Kneel on one knee in front of a chair or block, placing the heel of your other leg in front of the knee that's on the floor; rest your hands on the chair for balance but don't lean hard on it during the exercise. Curl the toes of the back leg under and stand up on both feet (figures 37, 38, and 39). With your hands remaining in place on the chair, check to make sure your feet point straight ahead and that one is directly behind the other. The hips should be square, heels down, and both legs absolutely straight. Contract the quadriceps of your front leg and lower the upper body over the front leg to feel a stretch in the hamstrings of that leg. Keep your upper body relaxed and breathe as you hold this stretch. There should be no pain in the back or hips. If there is, raise the upper body until the pain stops. Release the stretch by kneeling back down to your starting position. Change legs and repeat.

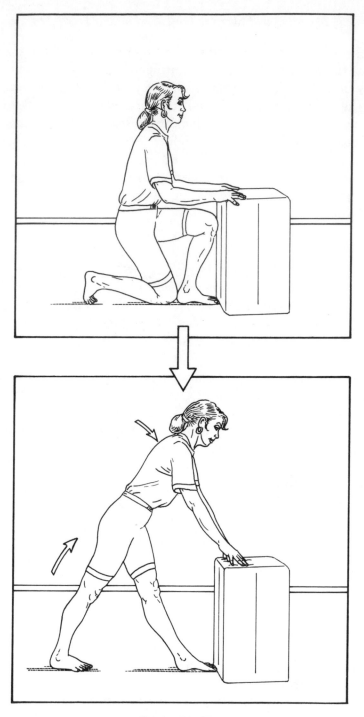

Figure 37–38
RUNNER'S STRETCH (MODIFIED)

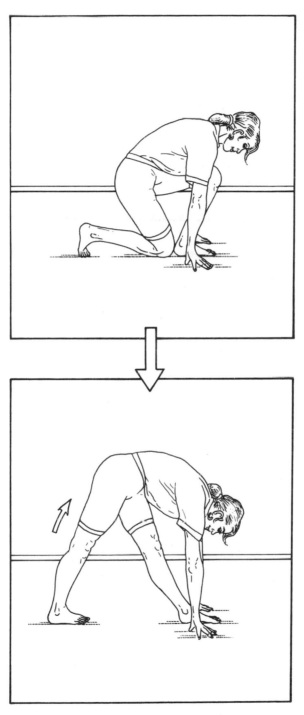

Figure 39
RUNNER'S STRETCH (REGULAR)

Spread-Foot Forward Bend
D-lux, exercise 16

Destination: We are stretching the muscles of the inside leg, the adductors, and stretching them from a stable pelvic position.

Route: (Hold 30 seconds each position.) Stand with both feet parallel and spread widely apart. Hook your thumbs together and bend forward keeping the back straight as possible. Touch the hands to the floor on the center-line of your body, keeping the hands even with the feet (figure 40). Hold for 30 seconds. Make sure the feet are straight, the legs are contracted, and the abdominals are pulled in.

    With the thumbs still hooked together, move your hands over to the left foot and hold for another 30 seconds. Remember, legs tight and keep breathing! With thumbs still hooked together, move the hands over to your right foot and hold for another 30 seconds. Return the hands to the center position again and hold for 30 seconds. Bend your knees as you come out of this stretch.

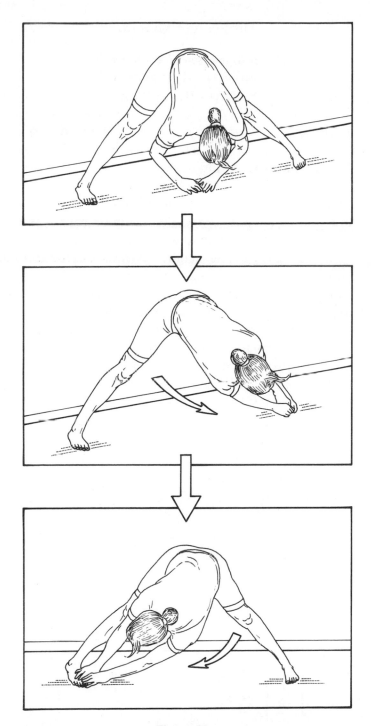

Figure 40
SPREAD-FOOT FORWARD BEND

Standing Quadricep Stretch
CONDITION II, EXERCISE 7
CONDITION III, EXERCISE 7

Destination: This is actually a hip stretch. We're doing it to activate the four muscles of the quadricep, which, in this case, is too tight. The hip is also reseating itself.

Route: (Hold 45 seconds to 1 minute.) Stand with the feet parallel and a shoulder-width apart. Bend one of your legs back so that you can place the top of the foot on a chair or block set behind you (figure 41). The height depends on the amount of stretch you feel in the quadriceps (thigh muscles). The higher the foot, the greater the stretch. Begin conservatively low and then go higher to find the right amount of stretch with no pain.

Keep your hips and shoulders square and tuck the hips under to feel a stretch in the quadriceps. You should hold onto something for balance. Keep checking to make sure the foot that's on the floor remains straight, and the hips are square and tucked under. Don't allow your back to arch as you roll the hips under.

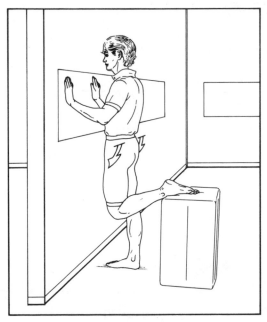

Figure 41
STANDING QUADRICEP STRETCH

Static Back Press
CONDITION I, EXERCISE 3
D-LUX, EXERCISE 21

Destination: Flat Hips, Colorado. We want the right hip and the left hip flat on the floor. If the Egoscue Method has a "silver bullet," this is it. It's our principle back pain–suppression exercise.

Route: (Remain in this position as long as needed.) Get down on the floor, lie on your back with both legs up at right angles on a block, a bench, chair, or bed. Your heels, calves, and lower legs, up to the posterior of the knee joints, should be resting on the surface of the block (figure 42).

Put your hands on your stomach or on the floor below shoulder level. Concentrate on breathing with your diaphragm. As you inhale, the abdominal muscles should expand, and as you exhale, they should sink. This rising and falling of your chest and abdomen must be visible, otherwise the diaphragm is not fully engaging. To get a feeling for what should be going on, rest a hand just below the rib cage. If it's not moving, inhale deeply and push with your abdominal muscles. Exhale and deliberately contract the abdominals.

Many people almost stop breathing while they are doing exercises. The gasping and grunting and desperation that set in during a rigorous workout are often the result of simple oxygen starvation. Breathe!

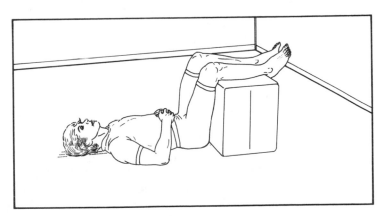

Figure 42
STATIC BACK PRESS

Let the back settle into the floor to allow the postural muscles to relax. Don't worry if your knees flop out a bit. After several minutes—exactly how long depends on the individual's dysfunctions—you will feel bones making contact with the floor. The arch in your lower back will flatten. Try to rotate your hips to the left and right. If there's no movement, the pelvis is on the floor where it is supposed to be. Don't bother trying to slide a hand under your lower back to see if there is a space; that just scootches the upper torso around in a misleading way. Try to determine whether one side of the body has settled in but the other is still up. Give it time to work. Initially, your kinesthetic sense will be dulled by dysfunction, however, it will soon start to tell you where your body is at any given moment.

The main purpose of the static back press is to relax the upper torso with the help of gravity. My business partner, Harland Svare, likes to take a nap while he's doing his static backs and it's a great way to listen to music or meditate.

This exercise may take thirty minutes (or longer) to get the back to settle down to the floor. Don't rush. If you are using the static back to suppress pain, and if the pain lingers, your back is telling you to stay down there and keep doing the exercise until it works—and it will work if you give it time.

Supine Groin Stretch
CONDITION I, EXERCISE 4
CONDITION II, EXERCISE 6
CONDITION III, EXERCISE 4 (SEE BELOW*)
D-LUX, EXERCISE 22

Destination: The hip flexors have forgotten how "long" they're supposed to be. We're reminding them, even though your shoemaker will hate me for all the lopsided, worn-out heels he won't be replacing in the future. The hip flexors, which lie along the inside of the thighs, are tough customers because they are designed to bear the full weight of the body. They can usurp the proper role of the quadriceps, and in so doing the knee becomes unstable. In effect, the hip flexors are saying "Knee? What knee? That's not my job." The quadriceps, whose job it is, can't intervene to protect the knee by operating the joint according to design because they've atrophied from lack of use.

Route: (Remain in this position as long as needed.) Lie on your back with one leg resting on a block, bent at a 90-degree angle, and the other leg extended straight and supported high enough to keep the back and hip flat on the floor (figure 43). One way to do this is to put a small stepladder beside the block or position the block just in front of bookshelves or the drawers of a dresser that are pulled out at various levels. Put your extended leg on one of the higher shelves or stepladder treads or drawers. (But keep the back and hip flat without actively trying to press them down. This is a passive exercise, so lay back and go along for the ride; the back and hip must settle on their own. If necessary, adjust the height of your extended leg—it may be pulling the hip and back off the floor if it is too high.)

Make sure both legs are in straight alignment with the hips and shoulders vertically. Prop the foot of the extended leg to prevent it from flopping to the side (everting). A pile of books will do nicely. After several minutes, lower the extended leg to the next level, making sure that your back and the hips stay flat to the floor, or just slightly off the floor.

Relax and breathe with the diaphragm. As the back settles into the floor, you will feel an easing of the muscular tension and strain, and when that happens, lower the leg once more. Repeat this process of relaxing the back into the floor as you lower the leg until your extended leg is on the floor. It should come down in

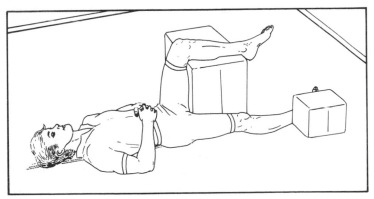

Figure 43
SUPINE GROIN STRETCH

three or four steps. (Each step could take 30 minutes or more depending on the severity of your dysfunction, but the more you do it, the faster the hip flexors will relax.)

If it's difficult to tell when the back is completely flat on the floor, another way of checking is to contract the quadriceps (of the extended leg) without any hip movement. If you get a good contraction in the middle and upper part of the quadriceps, the beefy portion of the thigh about halfway between the knee and the hip, then you have relaxed the hip flexors enough to allow the leg to be lowered to the next step down. But the hip should not be trying to help by twitching or rolling or pushing.

Make sure you (all conditions and D-lux) change legs and repeat the same process on the other leg. One leg always remains bent up at a 90-degree angle, so that both legs are *never* extended at the same time.

The purpose of this exercise is to soothe the savage beast—to relax the hip flexors. You may feel like you're not doing much, but the time spent in the supine groin stretch is very valuable. In fact, it's critical!

If you are a Condition III patient: this exercise follows the supine groin with towels, which is part of the towel sequence. Since your quadriceps will be contracting properly at the end of the supine groin with towel exercise, you'll only have to wait for your back to settle onto the floor after removing the towels. Plus, you do not need to extend your legs into the three raised positions. It is sufficient to keep the extended leg flat on the floor in the manner of the recommended technique for the supine groin with towels.

Upper Spinal Floor Twist
CONDITION II, EXERCISE 12
D-LUX, EXERCISE 14

Destination: The goal of this stretch is to get the hand, forearm, and shoulder to touch the floor. A really advanced stretch has the whole shoulder on the floor. Upper torso rotation is what we are after here. The shoulders and muscles of the upper back need to be given a refresher course on their full range of motion independent of what's happening in the hips.

Route: (Hold as long as needed. Most Condition II patients will need several minutes.) Lie on your side with both knees together and bent to form a right angle to your body. Extend your arms out, level with the shoulders, parallel to the bent legs, and palms together. Slowly lift the top arm up and over to the other side, turning the head to look toward the ceiling. Adjust this arm position to find the slot at the shoulder that feels comfortable to you. Breathe, relax, and let gravity slowly lower the arm to the floor.

Make sure the top knee does not slide off the lower knee. You may put your other hand on the knees to make sure they stay together. After the shoulders have settled as much as they are going to, come out of it by first inhaling and then exhaling while you lift the arm up and back to the starting position. Be sure that the palms match up and hold this position a moment before changing sides to repeat the exercise.

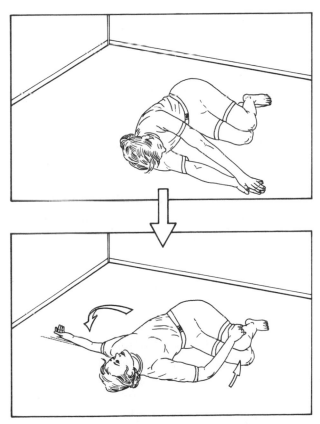

Figure 44
UPPER SPINAL FLOOR TWIST

Towel Sequence
CONDITION III, EXERCISE 3

Destination: Basically, we're headed the same place as in the static back press and supine groin exercises. But in Condition III, the muscles of the pelvic girdle, thighs, and lower back are so weak and dysfunctional, the purpose is to develop strength uniformly throughout the muscle groups. We have to do it while counteracting the flat, S-curve*less* back that comes with Condition III. Do A, B, C, D, and E as a complete sequence.

Route: A. Towel Static Back: You'll need two bath towels. Fold each one lengthwise, down the middle. Roll them end to end, jelly-roll style, but make sure both come out with the same circumference, about 9 inches. You may have to experiment with the towels to get the right circumference. The more severe the dysfunction, the smaller the towel; I don't want to impose an artificial arch in the back. In the clinic, we put patients with active back spasms down on a minimum of a 7-inch towel circumference; you probably won't need less than that.

Lie on your back, knees up, both feet flat on the floor (the heels and soles in contact with the floor and pointing straight ahead), with one towel under your neck and the other under the lumbar region of the spine just above the waist. Spend 3 to 5 minutes letting your back settle into the towels (spend more time if necessary).

B. Towel Knee-Pillow Squeezes: Keep the same position as in the towel static back. Widen your feet enough to accommodate a ball or a couple of pillows between the knees. Squeeze the knees together using the inside, abductor muscles of the thigh. Give the pillows a firm squeeze, then relax (but not enough to let the pillows slide out from between the knees). Do 3 sets of 10, and build to 5 sets of 15.

Make sure your hip muscles and abdominals aren't participating. If they are, you'll feel a contraction or tightening in the hips or tummy as you squeeze the pillows. That's not what we want. The object is to get the abductor muscles to go to work. The abductors move the limbs away from the median plane of the body. Adductors draw the limbs toward the median plane. To walk and run, when the abductors are functional—five of them work as a team on each side of the body—they tilt the pelvis toward the standing leg, allowing the free forward motion of the swinging leg. When it comes time to back up or otherwise change directions, twelve muscles participate in the adduction of the thigh. They are anchored to the pelvic girdle, and grouped in each thigh and buttock; the most powerful run along the inside of the thighs. Both types of muscles are weak in this condition, whereas in Conditions I and II the strong adductors have taken over.

C. Glute Contraction: Stay on the floor as in the first exercise in this series. "Glutes" is the shorthand name we use for the muscles of the buttocks, *Musculus gluteus*. It's easy to forget about them, but they're an important muscle group that, among other things, is vital in the proper vertical movement of the foot when we are walking.

Try to squeeze the glutes together; give them a good solid contraction on both sides. Many people have trouble finding the glutes. They're there. Keep trying. Sometimes it helps to touch your buttocks with your finger tips; the tactile sense assists in locating the muscles.

Squeeze, and squeeze equally on both sides. However, don't use the abdominals or pelvic muscles. Do 3 sets of 10, and build to 5 sets of 15.

D. Isolated Hip Flexor Lifts: 3 sets of 5; build to 3 sets of 20. Lie on your back with knees bent and feet flat on the floor, towels in place behind the neck and lower back. Lift one foot 6 to 8 inches off the floor. Keep the knee in line with the shoulder and the foot in line with the knee. Hold for a moment and return to the floor. Perform the designated number of repetitions in one set, and then repeat with your other leg. Keep alternating sets between legs until the designated number of sets is completed. Make sure you don't lift the knee too high. You should feel the hip flexors doing the work rather than the abdominals or quadriceps.

There may be some tightening in the lower back as each leg is lifted. What you're feeling is the hip flexor engaging at its origination point. We are promoting the ability of the hip to move laterally, and engaging the muscles of the back and buttocks.

E. Towel Supine Groin Stretch: Lie on your back with the towels in place (neck and lower back). Have one leg bent at a 90-degree angle and resting on a block or chair, while the other leg is extended straight and resting flat on the floor (the heel of the foot in contact with the floor). Prevent the foot from everting by bracing it with a stack of books or another heavy object (don't worry about the foot that is resting on the chair). Keep the back and hip flat without actively forcing them down. This is a passive exercise and if you start engaging your muscles it will defeat the purpose. If the hip and back aren't flat, adjust the towels or the height of the chair that you are using; it may be too high, which would drag the hip and back off the ground.

Make sure both legs are in straight alignment with the hips and shoulders. Relax and breathe with the diaphragm. As the back settles into the floor, you will feel an easing of the muscular tension and strain. At the same time, the hip flexor (on the side that's extended and resting flat on the floor) will relax and allow the quadriceps to engage properly.

If it's difficult to tell when this is happening, and it will be at first, contract the quadriceps slowly and without any hip or knee movement. If the hip and knee are trying to help out by twitching or rolling, the hip flexors need more time to relax. After a few more minutes try again and you will start to notice that the quadriceps is contracting in a progressive fashion as it (actually the quadriceps has five component muscles) moves up the thigh. There will be an obvious point at which the muscle(s) stops being taut and well defined. You'll be able to feel this with your fingers. The object is to have the solidity extend all the way up to the hip. Once you get a good contraction in the middle and upper part of the quadriceps, the beefy portion of the thigh between the knee and the hip, without knee or hip involvement and a well-defined quadriceps all the way to hip, then you have relaxed the hip flexors enough so that you can switch legs. Just reverse the procedure with the now-relaxed hip flexors and leg up in a 90-degree angle on the chair or block.

Make sure you always change legs and repeat the same process on the other side. One leg remains bent up at a 90-degree angle, so that both legs are *never* extended at the same time.

The more you do this exercise, the quicker the back and hip flexors will settle down and relax. In the beginning take your time and make sure the quadriceps is engaging.

Triangle
D-LUX, EXERCISE 8

Destination: The triangle is getting your lower back, hips, and thighs to work together without having any one group of muscles opting out or taking over.

Route: (Hold 45 seconds to 1 minute on each side.) Stand with your back to the wall, feet spread wider than the hips, and both feet straight ahead. Turn the left foot out to the side so that it is perpendicular to the straight foot (figure 45). Your right hip should not rotate in a counterclockwise manner; make sure your hips stay squarely on the wall. Drop the left arm down behind the left leg, and extend the right arm straight up to the ceiling with the palm facing out (as though you were waving hello or good-bye; your left hand, meanwhile, is lightly grasping the posterior of the left thigh). Look up at the back of your hand as you hold this position and breathe. Make sure both quadriceps are tight and abdominals are contracted.

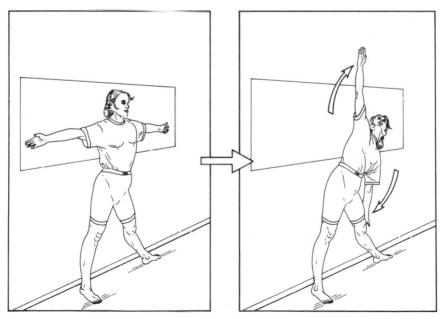

Figure 45
TRIANGLE

Remember you are bending directly to the side (left, over the hip and down), not leaning forward. Use a wall as a guide and keep your head, shoulders, and hips touching the wall throughout the stretch. There should be no pain in the back, but you should feel this in your inner thighs, quadriceps, and along the side of your body. Reverse the directions to repeat on the other side.

Under Air Bench
CONDITION III, EXERCISE 6

Destination: Unlike the air bench, this exercise is engaging the muscles from the hip to the shoulders, all of which need work.

Route: (Hold 1 to 3 minutes.) Stand against a wall with your hips, back, and shoulders pressing the wall. Place feet shoulder-width apart in front of the wall. Make sure the feet are far enough away from the wall so that when you bend your knees they are above the ankles, not the toes. Bend the knees and lower the body down the wall (figure 46). Push against the wall with your entire back and shoulders (don't forget about the lower back) to feel the quadriceps working. The strain should be felt equally in both the right and left thighs.

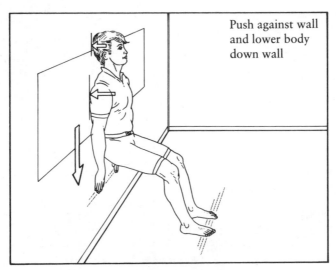

Push against wall and lower body down wall

Figure 46
UNDER AIR BENCH

If you have pain in the kneecaps, slide up the wall a bit. Do not bend knees to less than a 90-degree angle. Check to make sure feet stay straight and knees are in line with feet, rather than flaring in or out. Breathe! To come out of this, use your hands to push off the wall, and then walk around for a minute.

Exercise Sequence for All Conditions

Condition I	*Condition II*	*Condition III*	*D-Lux*
1. Arm Circles	Arm Circles	Arm Circles	Arm Circles
2. Elbow Curls	Gravity Drop w/ Scapular Contractions	Cats and Dogs	Elbow Curls
3. Static Back Press	Downward Dog	Towel Sequence	Cats and Dogs
4. Supine Groin Stretch	Runner's Stretch	Supine Groin Stretch	Isolated Hip Flexor Lifts
5. Abdominals	Frog	Foot Circles/Point Flexes	Cats and Dogs
6. Foot Circles/Point Flexes	Supine Groin Stretch	Under Air Bench	Abdominals
7. Cats and Dogs	Standing Quadricep Stretch	Standing Quadricep Stretch	Downward Dog
8. Downward Dog	Abdominals	—	Triangle
9. Runner's Stretch	Foot Circles/Point Flexes	—	Extended Lateral
10. Air Bench	Crocodile Twist	—	Push-ups
11. —	Pelvic Tilts	—	Foot Circles/Point Flexes

Exercise Sequence for All Conditions (continued)

Condition I	Condition II	Condition III	D-Lux
12. —	Upper Spinal Floor Twists	—	Quadratus Lumborum Stretch
13. —	Air Bench	—	Runner's Stretch
14. —	—	—	Upper Spinal Floor Twist
15. —	—	—	Cats and Dogs
16. —	—	—	Spread-Foot Forward Bend
17. —	—	—	Hip Crossover
18. —	—	—	Hip Lift
19. —	—	—	Air Bench
20. —	—	—	Frog
21. —	—	—	Static Back Press
22. —	—	—	Supine Groin Stretch

D-LUX: A TIME SAVER

I realize that a menu of 22 exercises may seem daunting. Many D-lux people just won't have enough time in the day to devote to the full routine. Here's an abbreviated menu that cuts a few corners while still requiring a full range of motion and design function: arm circles, elbow curls, cats and dogs, abdominals, foot circles/point flexes, downward dog, runner's stretch, upper spinal floor twist, cats and dogs, air bench, static back, and supine groin. The modified menu should take about 30 minutes to complete. Observe the sequence as I have listed it. For any of the moves that specify a bench, you don't need to rush out and buy one. Do the exercises on the floor.

6

Quiet Desperation, Quiet Hope

How am I doing?

Former New York City mayor Ed Koch tossed that question out so many times it became his political trademark. It's a good one; everybody in the service industry should ask it 100 times a day. And writing a book like this is pure service. There's no point if I'm not getting the Egoscue Method across to the one person that counts—you.

In my clinic it's easy to find out how I'm doing. I can see by looking at the patient, or he or she will come right up and tell me: "I don't understand." Then it's easy. I back up and try again.

Often, though, people are shy, or they don't really know that they don't know. In those cases, the best indicator is the way questions are phrased. I've pulled together several typical examples in this chapter. You may have a few of your own along similar lines.

Q: The daily grind is often stressful. Is stress a significant factor in back and joint pain?
A: Start with the basic premise that pain is a symptom. Now if you're having a bad day, with lots of things going wrong and high pressure decisions to be made, the pain in your lower back is not a symptom of stress. It is a symptom of dysfunction. What's happened is that on a "good day" the dysfunctional body has managed to cope; it suppresses the symptoms of dysfunction before

there is pain using whatever limited functions and compensating motion that are available.

In other words, the body tries to work around a dysfunction, but the route it finds is never up to the job for very long. The stressful situation comes along and overloads the compensating mechanism—the old straw that broke the camel's back. And there's pain.

Another important factor is that dysfunction, by definition, puts demand on muscles; they're either in contraction or flaccid, and as such they are being deprived of oxygen. When an additional episode of stress develops—a customer gets angry with you, the kids misbehave—it's just enough to nudge the dysfunction over the edge to pain.

Why? Instinctively our reaction to stress is to stop breathing. The gasp of amazement that we hear from a theater audience when the unexpected occurs is the sound of a roomful of people suddenly holding their breath. A hundred diaphragms freeze. In the office, when the customer cancels the order, the disappointed salesman does the same thing; the pain that he or she attributes to stress really comes from that extra hit of oxygen starvation on the dysfunctional muscles.

The body, by the way, needs stress. If a lab technician takes tissue samples, isolates the cells, and transfers them to a totally quiescent medium, those cells will die. Systematic application of stress is the way we train, learn, and grow. Without stress there is no stimulus. Torpidity, anger, depression, stiffness, and soreness set in as stress mounts because the individual is dysfunctional to start with. Great athletes are under great stress, but they're far from torpid or depressed or stiff. The most successful people in any profession are successful because they thrive on stress by way of their functional bodies.

Q: What about shoes? What should I be wearing every day? And what should I be wearing to exercise?
A: The less shoe the better in both cases. As long as your foot is pointing straight ahead, it doesn't matter what shoe you wear. The shoe manufacturers are selling shoes for dysfunctional feet— feet that are pronating, supinating, bearing weight improperly.

The shoe design masks the symptoms of dysfunction—or attempts to—and those symptoms move into the ankle, the lower leg (shin splints, etc.), the knee, and the hip.

There's a lot of criticism of sandals, but there's nothing wrong with them on a functional foot. An Ethiopian marathoner won the Olympic gold medal several years ago running in bare feet.

Q: Is there a point of diminishing returns when it comes to exercise and movement? I have heard that a workout lasting longer than 30 minutes is a waste of time and energy.

A: First of all, just moving—any old movement—isn't enough. I'm talking about design movement. Where people go wrong is that they decide "Okay, I've got to get back in shape." They start running or hitting the basketball court after years of being on the sidelines. By that point, the necessary functions are on "hold." To run or play basketball, the body starts compensating, using muscles and joints that weren't intended for the job. Pretty soon there's pain.

As for 30 minutes of exercise, it's ridiculous to think that the body has an internal stopwatch ticking away, and precisely at 30 minutes—not 29 or 31 minutes—says "Wait, that's enough." But the body does, in fact, know when it's had enough. It will tell you. More and more effort will be required to run or row or operate the StairMaster until the motion stops being pleasurable.

I'm not saying that it's time to stop when you begin sweating, working at it, and growing short of breath. There are plenty of pleasurable activities that require work, sweat, and wind—sexual intercourse, to name one of them. My contention is that by deliberately pushing an exercise past the pain threshold, we are simply engaging in a form of masochism which does not yield any real fitness benefits, and may in fact be injurious.

Q: How much movement is enough to maintain fitness and function? Is there a ballpark figure?

A: Motion, any motion in any amount, is better than no motion at all. But my previous answer applies here as well. Ideally, the movement should be design movement. As for the length of the workout, many patients would like me to say "You have to go at it 45 minutes a day without fail," or "In your case it's 62 minutes each Monday, Wednesday, and Friday."

It doesn't work that way. The pleasure principle is still the key determining factor. If I arbitrarily insist that a busy corporate executive spend 45 minutes a day exercising to maintain his functions, and if that guy can only spare 20 minutes, the full workout will stop being a pleasure and become a burden. In short order, he will stop moving, even though he knows that he should keep at it. That's why most fitness programs fail.

The Egoscue Method recognizes that the body knows best—not the trainer, not the theorist, not the aerobics instructor. It's a complete waste of time to try and tell the body to do something it can't do. All the talent, dedication, and ability to withstand pain are of no avail. However, by just starting the process, moving enough to remind the body of the pleasure it derives from proper movement, I can get the ball rolling; momentum will start gathering. If 5 minutes of motion was the outer limit, soon it will be 10 and then 20. The busy executive who said "no way" to 45 minutes will eventually find the time because he enjoys the 20 minute workout so much.

Q: Obviously, though, a 5 minute workout isn't enough, is it?
A: It might be. It depends on the individual's environment. If he or she is getting enough motion naturally, there is no need from a function standpoint to insist on imposing an exercise regimen for the sake of imposing an exercise regimen.

The paleolithic hunter-gatherer got sufficient motion from hunting and gathering. He didn't need a health club. When I watch TV documentaries on aboriginal people, I never see dysfunctional bodies: The shoulders and hips are square; the heads are erect and the feet point straight ahead. But at the margins, where civilization has begun to intrude on that primitive way of life, dysfunctions will start to appear. It's not at all unusual to see a sloping shoulder in an eskimo who uses an outboard motor instead of a paddle. The environment has stopped requiring the necessary motion to maintain his shoulder functions. Perhaps in the case of the eskimo fisherman 5 minutes would be enough to restore the function, but the rest of us living in "civilization" are going to need more than that.

Q: How much more?
A: Whatever it takes to restore the lost functions and to maintain them from then on. I know it sounds like I'm ducking the question, but I refuse to play the "one size fits all" game. One diet, one exercise program, one drug or surgical procedure does not fit all. That's why so many people give up on themselves. They try the miracle cure and it doesn't work. "Must be something wrong with me . . . I didn't have enough stick-to-it-iveness to jump around in front of the TV set with Jane Fonda for 30 minutes a day. I'm a real loser."

What I say to the people who come to my clinic is this: "How much time can you give me? Fifteen minutes a day, a half hour, an hour?" Whatever first pops into their heads is the right amount of time. Occasionally, somebody will answer "Whatever it takes." Then I may prescribe a routine that runs to 75 or 80 minutes a day, and those people will make rapid progress. It might take an individual who follows a 20 minute menu nine months to become fully functional. Those who are on the fast track—and on it because they want to be there—may get to the same point in three to six months.

Q: Can you tell by just looking at somebody how long it will take to get them back in the shape?
A: Yes and no. Yes, in that a Condition III person is going to take a lot longer than somebody with mild Condition I symptoms, like slightly everted feet and a minor hip tilt. No, because the Condition III person may be ready to take responsibility for his health, while the Condition I guy thinks it's the therapist's job to straighten out his hip.

Q: What about using a heating pad when you're in pain?
A: Trust your instincts. If the heating pad helps, use it. Remember, however, that the heat is not curing the problem.

Q: How about back braces; are they ever justified?
A: Not in the long run. The body works from the inside to the outside. The brace is trying to stabilize from the outside in, and it can't be done.

Here's an analogy: Would you reach under your car and try to grab hold of the drive shaft? I hope not. And even if you could rig up some sort of powerful device to clamp hold of the shaft, the result would be that the guts of the car would be torn out.

Like the gears of the car's engine and transmission, the muscles and joints are still working no matter what the brace is doing to the exterior of your body.

The brace gives you a false sense of structural stability and it overrides the body's mechanism for warning you, with pain, that you are doing things that will cause damage. That's what pain is there for.

A dysfunctional body that is hurting—I'm talking about chronic conditions, not the traumatic effects of a serious accident—has run out of redundant systems to use for compensating motion. The body is extremely ingenious when it comes to improvising its way around a problem. If I can't bend over using muscle group A, I'll use muscle group B; if I can't use muscle group B anymore, I'll go to muscle group C. Eventually, it's the end of the line, though, and the pain announces that fact.

In effect, you're being told "Stop!!!—before something really goes wrong." The brace encourages you to run that stop sign.

Q: Aren't drugs, particularly pain killers, justified in some cases?
A: Of course. With severely traumatic injuries, pain killers give the body a chance to stabilize and gain strength. We are really good at triage. Traumatic injuries that killed ten years ago are now survivable because of medical advances. But when it comes to chronic pain, the situation is not nearly as impressive, and pain killers are nothing but trouble. They louse up the body's internal communications network. The messages that are being sent out never get through.

Frequently, I have to negotiate a patient off a long list of drugs. They've forgotten which is which, and what each one is supposed to do. We play twenty questions: "How about this one?" I'll ask. "That's for cramps." "And this one?" "Headaches." In a little while we discover that the cramps started right after the headache medicine was prescribed. One by one, using common sense, we'll eliminate drugs that counteract or compound each other's effects. The client can go home to his doctor and say, "Hey, do I really need this?" And they can discuss it.

A pain killer relieves pain; it does nothing about the problem. A therapeutic program based on pain killing drugs is by definition a failure. It's treating symptoms, not the primary causes of the illness. And it's not just pain killers. I worked with a woman recently who was severely constipated. Her physicians had blasted her with every laxative and procedure they could think of. Nothing helped. She was Condition III and her pelvis was rolled under sufficiently to affect the bowels. No drug is going to take care of that. The constipation was a symptom of her dysfunctional pelvis. Every system of the body—colon, heart, lungs, stomach, you name it—is dependent on motion. If there's no motion, there's dysfunction: constipation, hypertension, emphysema, indigestion. And what happens? We reach for the Ex-Lax, the aspirin, the inhaler, the Maalox. We treat the symptom and wonder why we aren't getting any better.

Q: I suppose we can accurately call the Egoscue Method non-traditional medicine. Does that mean you are anti-physician?
A: What could be more traditional than respecting the design of the human body? But let's not argue semantics. If I find fault with physicians, it's this: Tinkering with a 10,000-year-old design takes a lot of chutzpah. And it also takes a lot of buck passing and complacency on the part of patients. Both sides are to blame.

But at least the patients often have an excuse: They're in pain. The physicians aren't. MDs are trained to see themselves as scientists, and scientists are the aristocrats of the white collar professions. Therefore, the patient is expected to suspend his or her judgment in the face of superior knowledge and social standing. When patients resist or question, they run the risk—real or imagined—of alienating the physician, which could mean continued pain and, perhaps, death.

Recently, a client told me that she had been treated by her physician like a "bored and crazy housewife" when she balked at continuing the powerful drugs that he had prescribed for her chronic jaw pain. The woman certainly wasn't crazy—she was hurting, as I could tell by observing the outward signs of her pain. Dysfunction and pain have recognizable signatures. They were written all over her; she was a classic Condition III. But to find the source of the pain, the physician either needed to spend more time with his patient—asking questions, listening to the answers, making observations—or he had to stretch his scientific methods beyond the boundaries set in medical school.

The "bored and crazy housewife" diagnosis was one physician's way out of a crushing dilemma. There are only twenty-four hours in a day, but physicians need thirty or thirty-five to handle their heavy workloads. To beat the clock, they use technology, either pharmacological or surgical. They can't reinvent the wheel for each patient, and as a result they rely on the expertise and research of colleagues who develop the latest generation of drugs and surgical techniques. Thus, technology—in this case, drugs—supplants the individual physician's judgment, judgment which would otherwise be shaped by interaction with the individual patient.

The phrase "reinventing the wheel" is most appropriate. Modern medicine is only about fifty to a hundred years old, depending on who is calculating. Even so, a mountain of scientific knowledge has already accumulated. The quandary of the doctor-scientist is that in addition, he or she faces hundreds of years of know-how, traditions, wisdom, and observations about the body that have not yet been subjected to rigorous scientific investigation. Therefore, this enormous mass of experience is of dubious value until it is proven with statistical certainty, using the tools that are acceptable to the medical-scientific community. Talk about a workload!

To manage, technology again comes to the rescue. What we know takes precedence over what we don't (scientifically) know.

The engineering problem of building an artificial joint is solvable. The deeper and more important question of whether the body's basic design will be violated by the joint is relegated to the file marked "To Be Researched Later."

I fear that by the time we get around to reinventing the body— and find that the design didn't need to be reinvented—it will be too late.

Q: Who's most at risk from back and other forms of joint and muscle pain?

A: Every man and woman with a white-collar job; every man and woman with a blue-collar occupation that requires them to stand in one place or sit for most of the day; every man and woman who commutes to work in a car, bus, or train; every child enrolled in school; every retired person who's told to "sit back and take it easy;" everyone who spends most evenings and weekends in front of the TV set; every Nintendo addict who begs for just "one more game, pleeeeease," after spending an hour only moving a wrist and forearm, head jutted forward and shoulders slumped.

Q: Is there something we can do at the office to counteract the lack of motion in the environment?

A: The best thing to do is to arrive at work in a fully functional condition and to stay that way. Beyond that, move around from time to time. Every thirty minutes, at least. When you sit still, the blood has a tendency to pool in your extremities. The oxygen flow to your brain, which depends on movement, is not as ample as it should be.

Breathing properly is very important. Slouching over a keyboard or leaning back in the chair impedes your respiratory system. And it's wise to avoid putting anything into your bloodstream that interferes with the red blood cells' oxygen-bearing capabilities.

I'm not a fan of soft drinks, with or without caffeine. Nor am I big on coffee and tea. There's nothing like plain old water. Dehydration is one of the secret troublemakers in the workplace these days. I'd say that less than 1 percent of the patients who come to the clinic for chronic joint and muscle pain are properly hydrated.

Almost everything in the modern home, workplace, and school environment is at war with the body's need to maintain adequate levels of fluid. The list includes central heating, air conditioning, overhead lighting, pressurized airplane cabins, and high salt content in food.

Most of the tissue in the body is composed of water. If it loses that water, the tissue drys up. The elasticity goes, and with it function declines.

Hydration and rehydration are important yet underutilized therapeutic tools. One sign of dehydration is lack of mental concentration—you can see it in a person's unfocused eyes and wandering attention. Someone who is in acute pain finds it extremely hard to concentrate and that same unfocused look is quite distinct. It's amazing how fast concentration begins to return when fluids are consumed. The patient's increased mental acuity can then be brought to bear on treating the dysfunction.

What's more, I believe there is a link between dehydration and pain. A compensating, dysfunctional body can be pushed over the edge to pain just by having to bear the additional burden of dehydration. The inelasticity of the body's tissues is what does it. While patients are in my clinic I insist they drink a lot of water— I'm a real pest about it—and often it's enough to give us a functional toehold to stabilize that individual's condition and begin recovery.

Q: Is it realistic to expect modern man to find the time and where-withal to move the way his ancient hunter-gatherer forebears did?
A: It's not necessary to spend twelve hours a day hunting and gathering to get sufficient movement to maintain the body's functions. But we do need to run our bodies through a full range of motion each day, and that's why I developed the D-lux maintenance exercises in chapter five. Without that full range of motion, function will be lost through disuse, just the way the car won't start if it's left sitting in the garage for several days. But the car, once it's jump started, will operate normally.

Unfortunately, our functions don't work that way. You just can't pull slumping shoulders back, flap them a little, and expect them to stay there.

Once we're functional, it doesn't take that much time or effort to maintain functions.

Q: What about people who can't move because of the pain?
A: "Can't move" situations are extremely rare. If dysfunctions brought on the pain, restoring function will eliminate the pain.

But we can't snap our fingers and expect those functions to magically reappear. I use the static back and groin exercises presented in chapter five to initially suppress the pain. The more advanced the dysfunction, the longer it takes, and the pain probably will come and go several times before it recedes to the point where it is no longer a problem. But if I can buy a person an hour of relief from what had been nonstop back spasms, that hour will rejuvenate him for the next step in the process. You win a small victory and you build on it.

Q: But can there be a final victory when you're dealing with something like slipped or herniated disks? Aren't those permanent without surgery?

A: No, not at all. The only thing permanent about a slipped disk or a herniated disk is when you don't correct the dysfunction that caused the problem; then it's a permanent dysfunction, isn't it? A Condition III individual, with his pelvis tilted under, has a weak upper torso and hips. Now if he starts doing a lot of heavy lifting, the muscles of the lower back, which are already under strain because the pelvis has flattened the S-curve of the spine, are being asked to hoist a fifty-pound sack of cement, in addition to keeping the spine intact—a job they can barely do in the first place because of the pelvis.

Something has to give, and it's the disk. That little piece of cartilage between each vertebra slides like a slice of cheese oozing out of a sandwich that's being squeezed too hard on one side.

The vertebra rides on that cartilage, tipping forward and back, side to side within the normal range of flexion/extension that the spinal column is designed to carry out. However, the dysfunctional pelvis is forcing the vertebrae to do some of the extra work of the muscles of the lower back. The extra work comes in the form of extra flexion which squashes part of the cartilage.

If we remove the dysfunction by getting the pelvis positioned properly, the disk will go back where it belongs. But a surgeon assumes the pelvis is a lost cause, or that nature intended it to be tilted under, and proceeds to go in between the slices of bread to remove the cheese because it's pressing on a nerve. But he can't just leave the bread sitting there without the cheese to hold the two slices together. Therefore, the surgeon uses his version of a big glob of peanut butter. He fuses the vertebrae.

If the cheese and bread simile seems simpleminded, think of the disk as a cushion or shock absorber that's being flattened in one spot and blistered in another. The blistered part is sticking out and bumping a nerve. The surgeon scrapes away at the blister and there's no more disk problem, at least not until our friend moves the next fifty-pound sack of cement with his dysfunctional pelvis. Another disk is now being flattened and blistered. Once again, a disk starts impinging on the nerve.

To prevent that from happening, after spending thousands of dollars in surgical bills, the hapless cement schlepper—all he wanted to do was build a patio—is told "Don't pick up any heavy objects."

It seems to me like that's an admission of failure. Go ahead and have expensive and painful surgery to fix your back, but it really won't be fixed after all. Plus, the solution is to restrict motion even more. "Don't pick up any heavy objects." Just what that dysfunctional person doesn't need—more lack of motion.

Q: Is it too late, then, for the person who has had a back operation, or a joint replacement?
A: It's never, ever too late. And the reason is that until the dysfunction is corrected, the problem which led to the surgery is present, still causing compensating motion somewhere in the body. The new knee may work like a charm. But what about the shoulder or hip? They are still under extra stress from the dysfunction. Just like a second disk rupturing months or years after surgery, there is an excellent chance that there will be another episode of pain, and that a surgeon will probably recommend another operation.

Many people come into my clinic and say "no way am I going to have another operation." They are motivated to look for an alternative, and the alternative was the only option in the first place.

Q: Okay, but the disk is gone, or there is an artificial knee. The design of the body has been changed, and that's got to make a difference. Doesn't it?

A: Not necessarily. The body has ways to adjust to the loss of the disk or to accommodate the new joint. And in many discectomy cases, the surgeon is counting on the remnant of the disk to reconstitute itself. Now, if the body is going to do that, why not correct the dysfunctional hip, or whatever, and let the disk mend itself?

I don't buy into the idea that these disorders are irreversible. Neither am I comfortable with the notion that since you've got one artificial knee that there's nothing to be done about your hip or your shoulder or your neck—you'll just have to have a second artificial knee.

There is something to be done. There is always hope. And I've got a perfect example. Last year, Jack Nicklaus noticed that as he played in various tournaments that there was one fan of his who was limping along from hole to hole following the match. He had a great deal of trouble getting around. Jack stopped play, went over to the guy and gave him my telephone number.

That individual, I'll call him Gary, came to the clinic. He had had a stroke three years before. Stroke victims, after they go through the recovery period, traditionally are given six weeks of physical therapy. At the end of six weeks the practice is to evaluate the patient's physical and mental functions to determine the extent of permanent damage. Once the evaluation is completed the patient is discharged with the understanding that whatever progress he made in the preceding six weeks, whatever functions have been revived in that period, constitute—more or less—the full extent of his recovery.

The therapists aren't heartless enough to say "go home, you'll never walk again." They encourage the patient to do what he can do. But usually the intensive therapeutic process is over.

For three years Gary gamely dragged himself around. The functions that were left were taxed to the limit and slipping away; he was slowly dying. When I saw him, I asked if he thought there was brain damage. Gary hesitated; he was reluctant to answer because he had been led to believe that the answer was yes. I pushed him and finally he said that he was convinced there had not been brain damage.

In return, I asked him, "Why can't you move then?" I wanted him to forget about the "stroke," just as I want other patients to forget their symptoms. The obsession with symptoms gets in the way of recovery. Gary needed to come at his dysfunctions as dysfunctions, not as STROKE.

We soon had him doing exercises from a static position—static back press, knee pillow squeezes, isolated hip flexor lifts—and he was seeing his functions engaging, and realizing that the "irreversible" stroke conditions that had been impeding his functions were in fact reversible.

There was an immediate improvement in his walking. The next day, I asked Gary why he couldn't open his hand, which was frozen in an almost classic stroke position, much like a claw that can't open. He shrugged.

I raised the hand and arm over his head and said, "Open your hand."

Gary opened his hand for the first time in three years.

There was still a lot of work to be done, but Gary knew from that point on that he was dealing with a problem that could be solved, not a condition with a scary name and a shelf full of textbooks telling him what he could and could not do.

Q: I don't have any pain. My back's fine; shoulders and knees have never been a problem. But after reading chapter four I realize that my feet do evert. It really doesn't seem like there's anything to get excited about. I see plenty of people with feet like that, including many professional athletes.
A: If you play a sport, you can significantly improve your performance by getting those feet back where they're supposed to be: Tennis, golf, biking, running, volleyball—I don't care what it is. If you're a skier, did you ever wonder why your turns and control suddenly go sloppy? Those everted feet are the reason why. Get tired walking? Feet. Wear out the outside heels of expensive shoes? Feet.

What's more, if you take a fall while skiing or biking, and your body is functional, there's less chance of injury because the joints are not making impact in a dysfunctional configuration. The situation is similar to a rubber band stretched to the breaking point. One more sudden pull and it snaps.

As for professional athletes, they're not immune to dysfunction. Many of them bring dysfunction to their sport, and fans will look at them and say, "Oh, right, I'll stand that way too. If it got him (or her) to the big leagues, it's good enough for me." Many champion athletes get to the top despite their dysfunctions. And they struggle hard against those dysfunctions to stay on top.

Finally, you mentioned the people we see on the street who show all the signs of dysfunction, but seem to manage anyway. You can't imagine how many of them are hurting. I'm reminded of Henry David Thoreau's comment, "Most men lead lives of quiet desperation."

7

The Games We Play

Now I'll ask you a question: What's your sport? If the answer is "I'm not into sports," it is time to figure out why that happens to be the case and what we can do about it.

In a world that requires motion for survival, participation in sports is irrelevant in an anatomical sense. The body gets enough motion to maintain its systems in the normal course of events. But we've established that motion is itself irrelevant these days, or seems to be, and thus sports are means to a very important end.

Sports gives us a rationale for moving by tapping into our competitive instincts, which closely parallel the subconscious and unconscious forces that drove our hunter-gatherer ancestors in search of food. As a therapist this competitiveness makes my life a lot easier. Without it, I have to invent something to persuade people it is fun to run, jump, twist, throw, stop, start, dodge, and sweat.

Eventually I'd have to invent basketball, probably the one sport that comes close to perfection: nearly the entire body gets a thorough workout, there's no gender barrier, the big bouncing ball is natural child's play, and for the elderly, why should shuffle board be the court of last resort?

One reason basketball appeals to me is that it discourages specialization. To play the game well it is necessary to be a generalist. These days, even the big guys have to scramble. Just standing under the hoop waiting for somebody to throw you the ball doesn't work anymore.

The game tends to reward those who are fully functional rather than "the Power House," "the Refrigerator," "the Mauler"—players with one or two highly developed skills or physical attributes used by coaches the way a grandmaster deploys the pieces on a chess board. Many athletes, despite multimillion dollar contracts, are walking catalogs of dysfunction. And that's why so many of them end up on the disabled list.

AN ANTIDOTE TO BOREDOM AND INERTIA

I'll address professional sports later in this chapter, but first I need to try and convince as many readers as possible that participation in sports can be an effective element in a complete fitness and therapeutic program.

Certainly, regular physical activity is a must. Solitary noncompetitive physical activities are fine. Almost any movement is better than no movement. But competition is so instinctive that it lifts mere physical activity to a higher plane, and once it's up there abundant motivation is supplied; usually more than enough to defeat the tendency to get too bored or too busy to keep running, swimming, cycling, or whatever else we've decided is the "right" thing to be doing to keep in shape.

Therefore, I'm biased in favor of competitive sports. It's a way to stay interested and stay honest. I love to rock climb, an activity that pits one man against one piece of a mountain. But I also run in ten kilometer road races to get a readout of where I stand against my peers. If I've been goofing off I know it after the first few kilometers.

No need to become a super-jock or a fanatic, but I'd urge you to rethink any aversion to competition: Is it because you're not the competitive type, or a reflection of something else? Perhaps an avoidance of confronting dysfunctions, not lack of skill or talent, that might prevent you from competing effectively?

NO HARM DONE

In choosing a sport, remember this: There's no such thing as a "bad sport." Some, like basketball, as I've mentioned, are better at introducing a full range of motion to the body. Others concentrate on the development of certain skills and muscle groups while neglecting others. None of them, however, is inherently harmful. (I'm referring to traditional sports. Bungee jumping is another matter.) The pain and injury blamed on a particular sport are the result of the individual athlete's dysfunctions.

The far right hand column of the chart (Table 1) proves my point. Anyone in the D-lux category can play the sports listed to the left without having their performance impaired by dysfunctions or encountering pain and other consequences of compensating motion.

Those in Condition III, however, have far fewer options. Out of twenty-four sports, there are only six that I would consider either moderately beneficial or falling into the category of offering no real benefits but unlikely to aggravate symptoms of dysfunction. The others? Forget them until Condition III symptoms have been eliminated.

I have also put Xs beside seven sports for Condition II patients, and four for those in Condition I. Don't take any chances. Don't think you are the exception to the rule. Playing through the pain sounds macho, but it is one of the dumbest things a professional or amateur athlete can do.

SELF-SELECTION

Runners and tennis players aren't going to like the news on lines 1 and 6 of the chart. In both cases, those with the symptoms of Conditions I, II, and III should temporarily retire until they've moved into the D-lux category. I'm not saying that they are guaranteed to start hurting, but the dysfunctions will take a toll on the body, which sooner or later will be felt. In the meantime, performance levels are, in fact, *certain* to suffer. All the hustle and dedication in the world won't change that.

Rowers and boxers should take heed as well—particularly boxers. A head that's forward and out of position, which is characteristic of all three conditions, is an invitation to brain damage. Serious rowers with shoulder dysfunctions risk rotator cuff tears and an assortment of repetitive-motion disorders. And dysfunctional hips can lead to knee, hip joint, and lower back problems.

Dysfunction and Sports

Sport	Condition I	Condition II	Condition III	D-Lux
Running	X	X	X	!!
Walking	O	O	X	!!
Track and Field	O+	O	X	!!
Gymnastics	O	O	X	!!
Cycling	O	X	X	!!
Tennis (racquets)	X	X	X	!!
Softball	O	O	O+	!!
Volleyball	!!	O	X	!!
Skiing (downhill)	O+	O	X	!!
Cross-country	!!	!!	O+	!!
Golf	O	X	X	!!
Baseball	O	X	X	!!
Football	O	X	X	!!
Basketball	O	O	X	!!
Soccer	O+	O	X	!!
Aerobics (high-impact)	O+	O	X	!!
Weight Lifting	O+	O+	O+	!!
Boxing	X	X	X	!!
Wrestling	O	O	X	!!
Fencing	O	O	O	!!
Rowing	X	X	X	!!
Swimming	!!	O	X	!!
Dance	O	O	O+	!!
Bowling	O	O	O	!!

Code:

X: avoid, not recommended

O: no real benefits, but not likely to aggravate the condition

O+: moderately beneficial

!!: very beneficial, highly recommended

Important note—None of these sports are inherently hazardous. However, no matter what the sport a dysfunctional athlete is a hazard to him- or herself.

Keep in mind that while we are all designed the same way, different circumstances can lead to variations in stress patterns. To avoid pain or incapacity, the body will find ingenious ways to work around dysfunctions. Condition II golfers, for instance, have astonishing tricks to compensate for their inability to transfer weight while swinging a club. There will be a series of little lurches, waggles, and twists. It's hard to find any two Condition II's who do the same thing on the tee—except hook, slice, and top the ball.

And those are the amateurs. By the time most professional golfers get to my clinic, years of compensating motion and the effects of hitting a couple of million golf balls make their lower backs look and feel like the proverbial Gordian knot (Alexander the Great used his sword to cut through the original Gordian knot and modern day physicians share the same impulse).

The chart helps explain why the idea has spread that there are good and bad sports. It seems easier to write off a sport than correct the dysfunctions. I know it isn't true, and I hope by this point that you do too. Yet, I'm afraid that is exactly what is happening. The chart indicates that in a dysfunctional world there will only be four big time participatory sports: softball, weight lifting, dancing, and bowling. All the others are headed for the "too dangerous" list.

The label has already been pasted on running. Thousands, if not tens of thousands of weekend joggers, have switched to other sports because they have been persuaded that running wrecked their knees or ankles.

I can tell there has been an enormous attrition rate among runners by simply flipping through old copies of the magazine "Runner's World." The pictures are striking. It's athletic Darwinism in action. With a pair of scissors, I can assemble an illustrated encyclopedia of dysfunctions: everted feet clopping along, a tilted pelvis jacking up a runner's hind quarters, a woman marathoner who seems to be traveling sideways because of her rotated hip and shoulders. But when I turn to current issues of the magazine, it is as though I am examining one of those "before-and-after" sequences. By and large, the dysfunctions are gone. The pictures are of athletes who look like they're in pretty good shape.

Now you could draw the obvious conclusion that runners are

better off today from a functional standpoint than they were ten years ago. You *could*, but don't be hasty.

The running craze has peaked. Fewer people are participating. The magazine pictures are showing us the runners who made the cut and are still on their feet, confirming that survival of the fittest, survival of the functional, is a pretty sound concept.

The dysfunctional runners have dropped out. Most of those who are taking part in ten kilometer races and marathons continue with the sport because it makes them feel good. They can do it. Their bodies are functional.

Running is a self-selecting sport. It selects *out* those who can't handle the demands, and selects *in* the ones who can. I know this sounds like stating the obvious, but many sports allow the participants to play through their dysfunctions. Lew doesn't jump very well in volleyball, for example, but he's quick and aggressive. If he stops short of becoming a volleyball junkie, playing seven days a week, Lew will probably never feel any pain or injure himself. Or if he does, Lew will blame his torn up knees on a fall he took on the ski slope the year before, or any other unrelated incident. He won't conclude that volleyball is dangerous.

What's given running a bad name is that runners do indeed become running junkies because it provides them with such enormous pleasure. When they're dysfunctional, the effects start to show sooner or later. Hence, running is "hard on the body," another hazardous sport. Thousands of words are written in newspaper and magazine advice columns every year about how to protect ourselves from the dangerous sport of running. The ultimate is to give it up altogether and bicycle or walk or take up high-impact aerobics, or better still, low-impact aerobics.

Before long, the health and fitness newsletters will be cautioning us to watch out for overdoing it on the bike and raising the possibility that walking isn't so good. High-impact aerobics have already fallen out of favor after only a few years of popularity. A recent report in the *New England Journal of Medicine* suggested that high-impact aerobics may cause neurological disorders.

Stripped of its pseudoscience, the logic, or illogic, of the case against high-impact aerobics goes something like this: "People complain of ringing in their ears and dizziness after a long, high-impact aerobic workout. All that jumping and twisting and turning isn't normal. The body is being asked to do something it shouldn't be doing. Ergo, high-impact aerobics may cause brain damage. There's too much concussion being transmitted up the spinal column to the skull."

Why is there an automatic assumption that the symptoms—ringing in the ears, dizziness—are symptomatic of human physical frailty? Let's use a little common sense here. If I picked up a novel written in French and turned to the first page to discover that I couldn't understand a word of it, my guess would be that I needed to brush up on my language skills. I wouldn't suppose that there was something wrong with the book, or the act of reading, to cause a sudden loss of the ability to comprehend French (particularly not if I couldn't speak French in the first place). Similarly, dizziness and ringing in the ears may be telling me that I need to brush up on my high-impact aerobic skills. Dysfunctional shoulders are as much a handicap to high-impact aerobics as a dysfunctional vocabulary is to learning French.

If children can spend half a day bouncing around on a pogo stick or skipping rope, why shouldn't an adult be able to twist and turn for half an hour? Vigorous movement and concussion, that is, jolting or bumping impact, in moderate amounts is really not that much to ask of a body—a functional body.

The symptoms we blame on high-impact aerobics or other sports are really symptoms of lack of proper motion. A head that is out of its proper design position—forward and down—is a head that makes the neck and upper spine muscles do a job they were not intended to perform. The muscles are there 1) to allow the head to turn to the right and left; 2) to permit the head to tilt up and down; and 3) to cushion the impact that is transmitted upward through the spinal column and the rest of the skeleton when the foot hits the ground. If the head slumps forward, the muscles go into permanent contraction to keep gravity from pulling the upper torso over into the fetal position. The head is a heavy weight balanced at the top of the spinal column, and once it starts to topple forward, the muscles can do nothing else but struggle mightily to stave off disaster. They lose the ability to function as shock absorbers.

The researcher who thought he was seeing high-impact aerobics causing vertigo and other neurological disorders probably did not notice that the subjects of his research were as dysfunctional as the general population. When they jumped and twisted and turned for half an hour, the concussion was indeed being transmitted to the brain. They were driving at high speed down a highway full of potholes without any springs, axles banging into the chassis, metal on metal.

What's more, those observed neurological disorders are valid symptoms. Like pain, they are giving us important information, not quit your aerobics class, but that the shock absorbers are shot! No matter whether an individual is turning somersaults or taking baby steps, there is impact every time the foot hits the ground. The body is designed to channel the impact, to make use of it by strengthening bone and cartilage, and to get rid of what's left over. When design-function is lost, the impact still occurs, although we may not feel it or know that what we are feeling is impact (dizziness, light headedness).

By recommending that people give up high-impact aerobics, the alarmists are actually urging us to, once again, censor the body's language.

ON TWO WHEELS

Many ex-runners have taken up cycling. It allows them to work out without worrying about things like muscle pulls and shin splints. In other words, they can ignore their dysfunctions. Even *Runner's World*, the bible of the sport, has taken to printing articles about how cycling can give runners a break from the punishment that's being inflicted by their favorite pastime.

But the punishment is coming from dysfunction, not running. Shin splints result when feet strike the ground improperly. Most often the runner is everting the feet. Thus, he or she is probably running on the outside of the heels instead of the balls of the feet. When the foot hits the pavement, it produces lateral torque that travels up the lower leg, chafing the muscles and producing the pain of a shin splint.

The dysfunction doesn't just disappear when the cyclist dismounts. His or her feet are still everted. Tired feet, sore ankles and legs, tripping, falling, hammer toes, calluses, bunions and corns are as symptomatic of dysfunction as the pain from shin splints while running. When you watch a cyclist pedaling down the street, look at the hips. The rocking side to side motion as he pumps first with the right leg and then with the left tells me there is a hip that isn't doing its share of the work. The rider is attempting to get a power stroke out of the dysfunctional hip by shifting his upper torso around and pushing down with it on the hip. He is using his back muscles and knees to propel the bike.

Another distinctive sign of dysfunction is a thigh and a knee that flares out away from the bicycle frame. The hips, thighs, knees and lower legs should be pointing straight ahead along a parallel line with the wheels of the bike. When the knee starts to point outward, that side of the body is taking a free ride.

Just like dysfunctional runners, dysfunctional cycling junkies will inevitably hit a plateau; their times won't improve, the extra mileage won't come as easily, there's pain here and there, and the sport feels more like work than play.

ON TWO FEET

"I think I'll take up power-walking," the ex-runner and ex-cyclist says to himself after his latest tumble into a clump of roadside shrubbery.

The bike goes into the garage, the new power-walker gets a set of hand weights and hits the sidewalk, still everting his feet, still dysfunctional in the hip, still rolling his right shoulder into the forward position. Well, I think you know what happens next. The power-walker isn't going to be at it very long. He's not getting the same kind of "high" he experienced running or cycling. If he goes out more than a couple of times a week, his back starts to kick up. He notices that his elbow and forearm hurt, the result of the hand weights interacting with the dysfunctional shoulder, a totally new symptom that he never noticed while riding the bike.

Power-walking sure is boring. What about swimming?

IN THE WATER

The perfect form of exercise. Or is it perfect because swimming ignores dysfunction? The ex-runner, ex-cyclist, ex-power-walker can chug back and forth in the health club pool without feeling any pain. He reaches the limits of his talent and capacity as a fish long before the symptoms of his body's dysfunctions reappear.

The reason the United States dominates international aquatic competition is that we have found a sport which does not penalize us for a motionless lifestyle. Many of our finest young athletes are taking to the water, realizing instinctively that they can excel in that environment. They feel secure and comfortable in the water because they are drowning out the body's messages of dysfunction. Unlike other sports, it doesn't hurt or make them feel anxious. Swimming feels good.

By counteracting gravity, a swimming pool allows the athlete to violate the body's right angles without being penalized. That's why physical therapists put their patients into the water whenever possible. It's much easier to move injured joints and muscles without a full gravitational load.

However, there's a slight catch. The body can't survive without gravity. Experience with space flight and extended periods of weightlessness have shown that our basic bodily systems start to break down in the absence of gravity. If you took a coiled spring and straightened it out, the properties that gave the spring its chief characteristic, springiness, would be lost. There would be no resistance. The spring would be just a limp piece of wire. The same thing happens to the body without gravity. It needs the stress and resistance that gravity provides. The relaxation-contraction sequence of the muscles is predicated on the existence of gravitational forces.

When people swim, they're not getting the full benefits of motion. The conscientious swimmer obtains an aerobic workout by doing several quick laps. He burns up calories (fewer than comparable nonaquatic activities) and moves many of his joints and muscles. But the body expects more than that from movement. For one thing, it needs impact. Just as insects have an antenna for reading their environment, we have a similar organ—it's called the foot. Every time our feet strike the ground, they give the body a readout, and the body adjusts accordingly. Swimming deprives the individual of his antenna. There is motion, but the body has lost one of its principle mechanisms for processing that motion and for energizing the systems in a coherent way.

Bone density is a good example of what I'm talking about. The foot striking the ground is really the equivalent of a sledge hammer whacking a slab of granite or a pile of sand. If you are holding onto the other end, your name doesn't have to be John Henry, the steel drive'n man, to immediately determine how much force will be needed for the next blow. You can feel it in your wrist, elbows and shoulders. In just the same way, the body assesses the continual interaction of the foot and the ground to adjust the amount of bone mass necessary to accomplish the physical demands that are typically being called for. This is a real "use it or lose it" process. The body does not waste energy building and maintaining superfluous systems. The body is, in effect, custom-made to operate in a given environment. In our case, as humans, the environment is *terra firma*.

What do you suppose it makes of all the swimmer's leg kicks, kicks without impact, and without a full gravitational load? In all likelihood, infrequent anomalous phenomena such as those, lasting twenty or thirty minutes at a time, may just be shrugged off by the body. Frankly, I don't know with absolute certainty. But my working assumption is that when it comes to maximizing the benefits of motion, swimming is not the perfect exercise that it's cracked up to be.

CROSS-COUNTRY SKIING

Concussion is one of the reasons that running is high on my list of ideal individual sports or physical activities. Cross-country skiing would be number one if it weren't for the lack of concussion (not a total lack because the heel does move in the binding). It forces the skier to move in an anatomically correct manner. The foot and the knee and the hip all go straight ahead. The upper body, meanwhile, gets a good workout, involving the arms and shoulders in the proper gait pattern with the legs.

A dysfunctional person can cross-country ski, but he will have to struggle harder with it. Fatigue will set in quickly and control will be limited. When I'm in cross-country ski areas, I notice the same pattern that I mentioned with runners. Cross-country skiing selects out the dysfunctional participants. When the sport first started attracting attention, people began to take part simply because it was something new. I used to see a lot of dysfunctional hips and shoulders and knees, but now those folks have decided that it's more fun to go to the weight room or use the nifty new stair-climbing machine at the health club. Again, what we see is survival of the functional.

ALPINE SKIING

Downhill skiing is a sport that many of its devotees fear has hit a plateau in terms of popularity. They worry that the soaring cost of lift tickets and equipment, warm winters in the eastern U.S. and Europe, and the aging "baby boom" populations are taking a toll. But injury and the difficulty of mastering downhill technique are also major factors. Both would virtually disappear if newcomers and veterans of the sport spent a little time correcting their dysfunctions before they got on the slopes.

A skier falls when he loses control, that seems obvious enough. But what isn't so obvious is that the loss of control, more often than not, is brought on by a dysfunctional hip which does not allow the skier to transfer his weight in a turn.

I can stand on the bottom of a ski slope and pick out the skiers with hip dysfunctions. They are the ones who are heading toward me, making classy, sweeping turns to the right and shallow, ragged turns to the left (or vice versa).

Ski instructors shout themselves hoarse at students to put weight on the downhill ski. But a dysfunctional hip won't take the weight. And those lopsided turns, and tumbles, when the ski tips cross the fall line and begin to gain speed, are the logical outcome. As he tries to turn, bringing the skis around until they are momentarily pointing straight downhill, the skier "hits a wall"—those skis won't go any further. So, he either shifts to his functional hip to check acceleration by abruptly turning the other way, or sits back on his heels on the dysfunctional side in an unsuccessful attempt to force the weight transfer.

Some skiers with hip dysfunctions compensate by skiing straight downhill! What little control they have comes from virtually skiing on one leg by making quick, bouncing, sharp turns. They'll also throw themselves into and through a turn, lunging shoulder-first and twisting the hips around.

Hot Dogger's heaven!

For a glimpse of hell, stand in the parking lot of a ski resort. Dozens of skiers with hip and foot dysfunctions will tramp by wearing their high-tech ski boots. They can hardly walk, and it's not only because the boots are stiff. The boots are forcing the feet to assume a *functional* position, and the hapless skiers go through incredible contortions to get to the lodge. That boot demands that the weight descend on the ball of the foot and refuses to allow the ankle to gyrate. It takes over the lower torso and leaves the skier, whose gait muscles are shot, to attempt to walk by using his shoulders and lower back.

On the slopes, the boots are holding the foot, knee, leg, and hip—the whole body for that matter—in the proper *functional* position despite the fact that the skier is dysfunctional. As a result, his joints, ligaments, tendons, and muscles are under tremendous strain. The last thing he needs to do is fall on them.

EFFORTLESS EXERCISE

The singles bar scene of the 1970s has evolved into the health club circuit of the 1990s. And that's okay with me. Any excuse or motivation is good if it results in more movement.

Here are a few tips for getting the most out of your health club.

The manufacturers of gym equipment are making and selling consumer products. They are continually refining and "improving" those products. But the improvement often takes the form of making it easier for us to exercise. The objective is exercise without effort; exercise without motion.

Consider the popular stair-climbing devices. The first generation was a real killer: no shortcuts, no mechanical assistance, all hip and leg muscle. It gave you an intense workout. But if your hip was dysfunctional, the workout probably only lasted about two minutes; anything longer was pure agony. The new Stairmaster, however, is a brilliant piece of work. It offers a modicum of mechanical assistance, an assortment of bells and whistles and, best of all, a little railing that allows the user to lean forward and swing the hip around and over the step to position it for the downstroke.

Wow. The railing makes the machine easier to use by providing leverage. People line up to get on the Stairmasters. The machine does not penalize us for our dysfunctions (use the Stairmaster at your gym, but lay off the railing).

But I guarantee you that there is no line for the rowing machines in the health club. Unfortunately, rowers are unpopular because they force you to operate in a functional position. The feet are strapped straight ahead, the seat holds the back straight and forms a 90-degree angle with the rail as it slides back and forth. The arms and shoulders must move according to proper right-angle articulation. You can't cheat a rowing machine, and they aren't used as much as other pieces of gym equipment that are more forgiving.

And what about those nifty weight machines sitting in every health spa window? They are a waste of time and money. Just ask any serious weight lifter. Here's why: Although billed as adjustable for each individual user, it's never exact. They don't acknowledge individual disparity or promote bilateral activity. Even though you can adjust the seat, it's hard to do and many people go ahead and use it the way they find it no matter how awkward the setup. Worst of all, the machines isolate muscle groups and take away reciprocal motion (although some of the newer designs are trying to address that shortcoming). Believe me, you're much better off with dumbbells.

The problem with weight training in general is that neither coaches, trainers, nor athletes understand the concept of bilateral function. They assume that if they execute the motion, the motion will take care of the strength problem. If the weight lifter has more trouble with one side or the other, they assume that's just his "dominant side." By this time you know there's no such thing. Many weight lifters also make the mistake of thinking they can get away with working from the outside in. They develop the peripheral muscles, the so-called "beach four"—the pecs, traps, biceps, and triceps—and forget about the inside muscles that are the musculoskeletal foundation. True fitness and function start on the inside.

TREADMILLS, TRACKS, AND TESTS

Of all the pieces of popular gym equipment, the Nordic Track is truly one of the best. It's glitzy enough to satisfy the craving for fancy gadgets and provide a thorough workout at the same time. The Nordic Track treats the body as a unit by engaging both the upper and lower torsos and the right and left sides of the body. The gym rats who use them are getting a balanced workout from head to foot and they really can't take any shortcuts or favor one particular muscle group over another.

Treadmills are also useful, but I'm not convinced by researchers and cardiologists who think they can use treadmills to accurately pinpoint an individual's cardiovascular capacity. Once again, we make an assumption as a tester or researcher that every given body, when provided the same stimulus, will react according to a basic set of patterns from which we can glean pertinent data. But they overlook an important point: If you put a functional individual on the treadmill and he uses his gait muscles, the big oxygen-demand muscles, his set of test parameters will be totally different than those of a guy who gets on the treadmill at the same speed, with the same set of stimulants, but whose feet are everted. There isn't any demand on his gait muscles.

Who has the better cardiovascular capacity? What is the true oxygen utilization capacity of Joe Duckfoot? What happens to his cardiovascular capacity when he suddenly has to use his gait muscles on a narrow stairway? The results with the treadmill stress test are not as exact as we think. Our data will be incomplete until we factor in functions and dysfunctions.

THE PHYSICS OF TENNIS

Tennis players are fun to work with and are they ever predictable! When their games start falling apart, they get a new racquet or a new pair of shoes.

And then we come full circle when their shoulders, knees, and elbows start hurting. "Must be my new racquet . . . must be the new shoes."

It's not the racquet; it's not the shoes.

"My concentration is shot," is another favorite second guess, "that's why I'm blowing matches." There are many excuses.

As soon as the wide-bodied racquets were introduced several years ago—they were just showing up in the sporting goods stores—I heard "the wide face on this new racquet of mine is aggravating my tennis elbow."

"It is?"

"Sure, the shock of the ball striking the wider face of the racquet is sending more vibration up the handle into my arm and elbow."

"Do you suppose that's why your right shoulder is higher than the left and rolled forward?"

"Well . . ."

"You haven't had that racquet for more than two weeks. It took you twenty-five years to get your shoulder into that position. The elbow is hurting because of your shoulder."

Serious tennis is very unforgiving toward dysfunctional bodies. To understand what's happening anatomically in the center court at Wimbledon you have to remember that proper weight transfer, which is essential in all sports, can only be accomplished from a balanced position. Dysfunctional tennis players, by definition, are unbalanced. They are always hitting off the back leg; the weight transfer, instead of going from right hip to left hip, is torquing wildly through the upper torso with every forehand and backhand stroke. In the days of the old wooden racquet only the very best and totally functional tennis players could get pace and put top spin on the ball because they were the ones who were balanced and transferring their weight properly. Today's high tech racquets are so sophisticated that you can get top spin and pace without being anatomically functional.

You also get hurt. And the reason for this is found in a simple law of physics—for every action there is an equal and opposite reaction. It's that equal and opposite reaction which is supposed to be happening in the equal and opposite other half of the body that is running amok.

When Mary came into the clinic a few years ago she was a fanatical amateur tennis player, but she was suffering from tennis elbow. She had tried every cure, including acupuncture, and would have had surgery except she was concerned that she would miss an entire season recuperating.

"Stand up for a minute, Mary," I said as I came around from behind my desk. She got to her feet and faced me. "Point your toes inward as though you were pigeon toed," was my next request.

"Squeeze your shoulders back—not up—back."

"Tennis elbow, eh? Hurts like hell, right?" I said. Mary nodded. I reached over and squeezed her sore elbow. Mary's jaw dropped. I squeezed it again. The pain that Mary had been living and playing with for months was gone.

Mary couldn't believe it, and she started poking the elbow as though the pain was in there hiding. I think she was a little miffed that it was gone.

I told Mary that by standing pigeon toed with her shoulders back she was proving that the hips and shoulders are a unit. "In that position, we are able to get some ball and socket function back in your shoulder. When the shoulder is forward and you ask for a ball and socket motion, like a forehand stroke, it can't deliver unless the elbow is involved. The elbow, which isn't designed for a ball and socket function, is nonetheless doing the work of a ball and socket joint. The contortions are snagging the tendon as it comes through the elbow."

One of the exercises on Mary's menu was gravity drops with scapular contractions, which she tells me she now uses at parties to wow any of her tennis pals who are complaining about tennis elbow. She takes them to a staircase and has them do three sets of twenty contractions, and then gives them a replay of my lecture on the ball and socket versus the hinge joints.

GOLF: THE HUNCHBACK OF PEBBLE BEACH

Golfers are just as bad—probably worse—than tennis players when it comes to blaming their dysfunctions on equipment or technique. They'll buy anything to shave a few points off their score. But golf is the one sport that has totally ignored the body. According to the gospel of the fairways, talent and technique, practice and perseverance, concentration and determination, make all the difference between salvation and damnation, the righteous and wretched. As a result, the locker rooms of the major tournaments look like sports medicine clinics. So many touring golf pros are hurting that the healthy athletes are the oddities of the game.

Unlike football players, golfers suffer in silence. There are no spectacular smashups on the back nine. But they are still suffering.

Like football and running, golf is eventually going to start being blamed for all the pain. It's inevitable, given the boom which has made golf the fastest growing sport in the United States. Sheer numbers alone will expose the sport to the same forces that transformed running from a largely invisible pastime for a small minority into a recreational activity for the masses, and which stopped just short of necessitating a surgeon general's warning on each pair of running shoes.

Many new golfing enthusiasts are coming to the sport for all the wrong reasons. It seems more like a social activity than an athletic event, an easy way to get some exercise and fresh air, relieve stress, and have fun. However, golf is athletically and physically demanding. The idea that golf is a middle-aged safe haven for the sedentary is nonsense. Anyone who expects to play without embarrassment and acute frustration has to devote a considerable amount of time and effort to mastering the basics. Once that process is underway, the new golfer comes face to face with his old dysfunctions.

"I took up golf after I wrecked my knees running," is a statement that should scare the hell out of anyone who loves golf. Golf does not tolerate dysfunction. That's why so many professional golfers are playing in pain. They bring dysfunction to the game—golf has nothing to do with it—and by playing hour after hour, day after day, the repetitive compensating motion gets them.

Unless golf faces up to the indifference it has traditionally shown to the body and its proper functioning, the booming interest in golf won't last. The sport will be swamped in pain. Twenty, thirty, and forty year olds who are now heading for the fairways in droves are the least functional generations that have ever teed up a golf ball. The very fact that they are interested in golf is worrisome. It suggests that golf is becoming the sport of last resort. Actually, the sport of next-to-last resort. The last resort is no sports at all. After an enormous investment building new courses, teaching facilities, and product lines, golf could end up bankrupting itself if today's newcomers become tomorrow's dropouts.

The quality of golf instruction these days is magnificent. I can't think of another sport that is taught as well. Even a modest goal like making the average weekend golfer reasonably proficient at the game—and golf is a demanding athletic event—is a major feat. The videos, instruction books, magazine articles, and one-on-one coaching are incomparable. All the more so because many golfers cannot even begin to do the one thing that's necessary to play a consistent game of golf—transfer their weight.

Extremely resourceful and adept instructors have managed to concoct various ways around the problem. The student may hook or slice occasionally, or lack power, but his game isn't all that bad. A dedicated golfer who is determined to make progress can go to the driving range and "groove" his swing by hitting buckets of balls. However, when he gets under pressure the groove disappears. And he thinks that his technique was faulty, but it's not technique.

The problem is stress: Stress eliminates learned behavior. By learning the technique for managing his poor weight transfer, the golfer (and any other dysfunctional athlete for that matter) seems to be getting along just fine, until he is forced to blast out of a sand trap to save his par. The inability to transfer weight comes back with a vengeance.

When their livelihoods are at stake, professional golfers are very resourceful. They'll work around the pain by adjusting their games, spend hours practicing a new stance or swing, and go roaring into a tournament like the second coming of Bobby Jones only to blow everything on the last three holes as the pressure mounts.

Before she came to my clinic, a young woman who plays on the junior LPGA circuit was having severe lower back spasms. In desperation, she went to Japan for treatment from a specialist who realigns and manipulates nerves. The guy did wonders. She felt great and was able to practice without pain for the first time in months. However, the night before her first big tournament the back spasms resumed.

Stress: The one thing the Japanese specialist couldn't eliminate. Her hip knew it wasn't able to really take the weight of the backswing. When practicing, she finessed it by compensating with other muscles and, therefore, the symptoms were absent. As the tournament approached, instinctively she began to swing in the only way that was really comfortable—that is, effective—reawakening the spasms.

Dysfunctions cannot be overcome with technique or technology. This goes for pain as well as performance. Many if not all of the skill deficiencies that plague the recreational golfer come from readily observable and correctable dysfunctions. If both sides of the body are not doing the same thing, it is impossible to have a symmetrical golf swing. Power, balance, weight transfer are all dependent on proper function. Try pulling your right shoulder forward and down, while pushing the left shoulder back. Now, put your hands together as though you were holding a golf club, preparing to drive the ball down a fairway. Bring your hands and arms into a backswing, but keep the shoulders where they are. You probably feel like the Hunchback of Notre Dame, and you'd have to go through extreme contortions to get the club face to intersect with the ball.

Today's golf instructors, bless 'em, could teach the Hunchback of Notre Dame to control the contortions well enough to get around Pebble Beach or Doral. But unless we begin to pay attention to the design of the body and its dysfunctions it won't be long before we hear how golf tore up poor old Quasimodo's back and left him limping around the belfry of a tourist attraction in Paris.

PROFESSIONAL ATHLETES AND DYSFUNCTION

Most of the professional athletes who come into my clinic the first time are in trouble. Not only are they hurting, but the panic of impending unemployment can be spiritually crushing. At the same time, though, they are very motivated, not only to stop the pain but to restore their athletic ability. Even so, it's a battle to make that champion tennis player or golfer realize that all the lost matches and the prize money that slipped through their fingers is as symptomatic of dysfunction as the excruciating pain they feel in the lower back.

The best athletes know intellectually and instinctively that they must control all the variables of their game. That's why they practice constantly. Great basketball players often have a favorite spot on the court, and as hard as the opposing team tries to keep them away from the spot, they'll get there, shoot, and score. There's no defensive combination that they aren't ready for. The variables are under control.

But the same basketball players are surprised to discover that their bodies have become a variable and they are not in control when dysfunctions set in. All the talent and experience and dedication in the world aren't enough.

One of the things I tell athletes, especially football and basketball players, is to look at their opponent's feet, knees, hips, and shoulders. A football lineman with a hip dysfunction, for example, cannot drive forward as hard and fast as a functional player. The same goes for basketball players. If their right foot is everted, they can't move to the left. Therefore, if you're playing opposite the guy, you should always drive to his left side regardless of whether he is left or right handed. The dysfunctional side doesn't have the strength to propel the player in the opposite direction.

These dysfunctions have serious implications for professional sports. Athletic excellence cannot be maintained if the individual players are physically incapable of performing skillfully and *safely*.

We're kidding ourselves into thinking that this generation of National Football League players can tackle or block properly. There's innate talent, dedication, and lots of guts, but they can't do the job because, with few exceptions, they are not functional. The coaches are the first to admit there's a problem. Their athletes are frequently sidelined by injuries, and the healthy ones aren't able to handle drills that were commonplace fifteen or twenty years ago. They cannot do simple things like a linebacker balancing his weight on the balls of the feet and driving forward without first bobbing upward to engage the hips. (That little bounce or bob is murder; it costs the player a crucial fraction of a second and makes him vulnerable to being hit and injured by the opposing player.)

The standard answer is to yell at the players and make them keep practicing, which of course is a waste of time since they can't possibly practice away hip dysfunctions. The hamstrings, glutes, and quads are not engaging because the hip flexors have taken over.

TECHNOLOGY SUBSTITUTES FOR FUNCTION

I'll give you an example of another functional deficiency that's as common as a seven figure contract for first-round draft choices. Try this: Hold your arms up and extend them straight out to the right and left level with the shoulders, palms down and parallel with the hips. You're going to do arm circles, so make the golfer's grip: Bend your fingers at the knuckles and point your thumbs straight ahead. Pull your shoulders back and make small circles with your arms by rotating them clockwise. Do it twenty times, and make sure your arms and shoulders remain parallel with the hips.

Arm circles aren't a real big deal if you're functional. But if you aren't, arms circles are tough. Could you do twenty? Did your arms and shoulders stay back like the wings of an airplane? If the answer is no, congratulations! You're a prime candidate to play for an NFL team.

Most pro football players (and many college players) have trouble doing arm circles. I ask players who come to see me to do a few and they say "Arm circles . . .? Sure thing." But what I get are arms that come forward like the handlebars on a bike. "No, Big Guy, out to the side. Pretend you're a bird." He strains to pull them back, and the elbows bend; those arms aren't even close to parallel with the hips. "Pull 'em back, Champ."

"They are back."

"No, they're not." He can't do it. His shoulders are locked in the forward position because the coaches have fallen in love with weight training. The romance began as a way to build strength and get an edge on the competition. Pretty soon everybody was doing it simply because everybody else was doing it. The fad spread through the NFL and down into collegiate and high school ball without much thought being given to the disadvantages. One question that needs to be asked is this: Why is it necessary to take the players off the field and put them in a weight room to build strength and speed, whereas a generation ago they developed plenty of strength and speed playing and practicing the game? And this is my answer: Those players came to the game functional; these players arrive dysfunctional. Their lack of strength and speed, and inability to develop them under traditional training methods, are manifestations of the dysfunctions; until they are corrected, weight training will only make things worse. Why are teams recruiting on the basis of their sophisticated training systems, rather than what happens out on the playing or practice fields? The coaches are trying to substitute technique, technology, for functional athletes.

Also, while we're examining this issue, we should ask if there is a correlation between weight training and the rising curve of injuries. When I look at the guys in the NFL and the difficulty they have with arm circles, my answer to that question is yes. Functional shoulders have tremendous flexibility to allow the upper body to twist and turn and adjust suddenly. The athletes have been robbed of their upper-body flexibility.

There is nothing wrong with weight training per se, but it has to be offered in a balanced program that recognizes the body's bilateral functions and unitary design. By going overboard with things like "power lifts" and "cleans" the athletes are being ruined. Now we have a league full of linesmen who are unable to block or tackle by putting their arms out to the right and left, without first twisting at the hips or turning their whole body by shifting the feet. Behind them, waiting for a shot at the big time, are the next generations of college and high school players, with dysfunctional, battering ram shoulders and heads pulled down and forward, just like their role models.

Nice work. Thanks to misguided weight training, backing a tractor trailer around in a full circle is easier than tackling a guy who is running down the field with a football. Here's what happens in the weight room: To get the barbell off the mat, the athlete hunches over and rolls his shoulders into the forward hinge position, which he thinks will give him maximum lift. He does it over and over again. After a while, the shoulders get the message— that's where we're supposed to be, forget all about the ball and socket. Try it yourself. Bring your shoulders way forward and down. You can feel the strain across the middle of your back. Try to turn to the right or left. See what happens?

Your upper-body flexibility is reduced to about zero. The hips must do all the work, and they share the increased burden with the knees. I wonder where all those knee injuries are coming from?

FASTBALLS AND CURVEBALLS

Every August when major league baseball starts showing its dysfunctions, we hear and read about how a pitcher's shoulder socket just can't take the strain of firing a fastball over and over again.

Really? How come Dizzy Dean pitched back-to-back double headers? Simple, Dean had functional shoulders and hips. A dysfunctional shoulder can't take the strain; it transfers the rotational stress of the throwing motion into the elbow. Compensating motion also takes place across the upper back around the rotator cuff and down in the hip.

If you watch the "aging" Nolan Ryan pitch, when he delivers the ball, his hips are square with the plate. The weight is transferred smoothly from hip to hip. His feet point straight ahead. It's the primary reason he is still pitching, despite all that "aging."

By ending up looking like a dog trying to run across the surface of an icy pond—a leg over here, a leg over there—most of Ryan's colleagues are throwing the ball by isolating a few muscle groups and making them do all the work, instead of using the entire musculoskeletal mechanism from head to foot.

To make matters worse, pitchers and their trainers forget all about bilateral design. They spend years developing their unilateral functions. The throwing arm, and that side of the body, become the equivalent of a 900-pound Siamese twin attached at the backbone to his 90-pound brother. Furthermore, the designated hitter rule in the American League eliminates the need to adopt a balanced and bilateral training regimen. Swinging a baseball bat is not easy with only half a body and, since pitchers are traditionally poor batters, the designated hitter rule was adopted in the first place because it was easier than going to the trouble of developing the whole athlete.

Baseball isn't on the "dangerous sports" list, yet. But it is edging in that direction; an ironic and ominous fate for a sport that calls itself America's national pastime. When I look at the sports and dysfunction chart (Table 1), it concerns me that we may end up with a bowling alley or an Arthur Murray dance studio as our field of dreams.

8

Modern Maladies and Our Children, Our Elders, and Ourselves

There's been an interesting experiment underway for about the last ten years. We're using our children as the guinea pigs and the results are just starting to show up.

What we're seeing is an answer to this profound question: Can children do without motion?

By "do" I mean develop physically and mentally, and lead fulfilling, healthy lives.

Based on my observations and the evidence I've accumulated in the clinic, the prospects aren't encouraging.

WITHOUT FOUNDATION

Mankind has been losing momentum for most of this century, and the phenomenon of motionlessness probably started with the onset of the Industrial Revolution. But today's children are members of the first generation to grow up in an environment that has been stripped of all but a few remnants, relics of the full range of motion that was once a normal part of everyday life.

As a result, most children never lay down the foundation they need to support essential physical functions. The process of building a solid functional base starts when the child is still an infant.

By twisting and turning belly down, then rolling onto its back to wiggle and stretch, the baby introduces its body to the nourishment of motion. As strength and coordination develop—movement begetting movement—it's time to crawl, giving hands and knees and shoulders and thigh muscles their first workout. Mobility leads to confidence and the desire to travel further and faster. Soon the infant is standing on two feet.

His or her days are filled with toddling, running, falling, jumping, and dancing; the child is establishing a full range of motion. Spend a few moments watching a pre-kindergarten group at play. The pint-size whirling dervishes do things with their bodies that adults wouldn't dream of trying.

But wait—those children have exactly the same design as an adult. The difference is the kids haven't lost the necessary functions. They are in the process of developing them as fast as possible (I hope).

Ian is swinging from the bars of the jungle gym. His hands are over his head and he is imitating a monkey. Gillian is pretending that she is a doughnut by leaning way over to her right side and holding onto her ankle.

When was the last time you, Dad, had your hands over your head bearing weight? And Mom, tell me when it was that you last bent at the hips laterally? We have elaborate mechanisms for performing those functions and we don't use them. But our children, if they are developing properly, are joyously and exuberantly using their bodies according to design.

If they are developing properly.

If their environment continues to encourage movement.

If . . . if movement is rewarding and relevant.

BABY SHOES

A couple of years ago, I was conducting a clinic at a country club in Westchester, New York. Toward the end of the day a young man and his wife dropped in. They were there to pick up his parents, who were participating in the session. Frequently, I get all the different generations from the same family as the word spreads about the Egoscue Method. In this case, the young man had attended an earlier clinic and was a real convert. David was totally committed to taking responsibility for his health. He had convinced his mother and father that there was no reason why they couldn't do the same thing.

The couple, as it turned out, had their infant daughter with them. I was standing in the back of the room fielding questions when they came in. I don't know whether David planned to do what he did or if it was spontaneous, given the presence of his little girl during a discussion of the benefits of motion. But in any event, he spoke up and I immediately heard the unmistakable tone of a worried father. He was nonchalant about it. David said he was wondering whether there was a problem with the child. He and his wife had noticed that she couldn't crawl.

"I don't understand," I said. "She can't crawl?"

"Well, we put her down and she starts to go, but then stops and cries. I think there's something wrong. Maybe we should see a physical therapist." David mentioned the possibility of "retardation." His voice dropped almost to a whisper when he said the word.

The mother was holding the infant in her arms. Now, remember, Westchester is no poverty pocket and the setting is an affluent country club. The child was beautifully dressed. A cute little thing. She was wearing very expensive baby shoes. Obviously money was no object for the family.

"Take off her shoes," I suggested, "and put her on the floor." There was silence as the group watched Mom and Dad untying the shoes. Uncertain about what to do next and probably a little anxious, the couple paused and looked at me for instructions. "Just put her down," I said.

The little girl sat there on her bottom for about ten seconds looking around at all sorts of interesting and wonderful things—chair legs, shoes, and gym bags that were just crying out for close inspection. She rolled over onto her hands and knees, looked up at her mother, and then zoomed off across the room. A baby with important work to do!

So much for the little girl who couldn't crawl. The expensive, soft-soled baby shoes were immobilizing the child. She couldn't get the necessary traction to crawl. She had been slipping and sliding. There are ten tiny toes attached to the two feet, and they have a simple but important job. They dig in so that the muscles of the foot and leg can push off. It was frustrating and too much effort with the shoes on, and, as a result, the child would sit there and cry.

I can imagine what would have happened if a physical therapist or a child psychologist had gotten their hands on that baby. There would have been a battery of expensive tests. Eye-hand coordination, balance, motor control—you name it. They would have had her wired up to check brain wave functions. How about her inner ear? Meanwhile, the baby would not be crawling and would not be developing. Months later, there would be a little girl who, because she wasn't crawling, would be slow to walk. Her confidence, curiosity, and energy levels would all be affected. She would cry a lot and have temper tantrums.

All because of a pair of baby shoes, expensive, state-of-the art baby shoes. I should have them bronzed. Like so many other kids, the little girl's parents were giving her the best physical dysfunctions that money could buy.

The human foot was designed to function *au naturale*—naked, bare. We don't improve on the design by putting it inside a shoe. On the contrary, by restricting movement shoes interfere with the design, and if the interference comes early enough in the developmental stage, a child can be deprived of functions before they have first manifested themselves.

Let me put it in another more direct way. Our children are becoming dysfunctional at a younger and younger age, to the point that many functions never develop in the first place.

The foot is a very good example. The arches of the foot distribute weight and participate in the balancing process. The arches—there are three of them—are maintained by muscles in the sole of the foot and the lower leg. As the arches change in tension, the muscles automatically contract and expand in adjustment. If the foot is enclosed in a hard shell, which is what the shoe is, you have altered the way in which the skeletal arches are free to react to tension. And because the body is a unit, the effects of this alteration are felt in the knees, the hips and the shoulders. Compensating motion sets in throughout the unit.

The superior ankle joint—the point at which our foot seems to join the lower leg—must function under what amounts to three and a half times the body's weight when walking. If the ankle joints cannot develop strength and flexibility because they are trapped in high-top baby shoes, which inhibit a smooth front-to-back movement of the joints—heel and toe, heel and toe—the normal gait or walking pattern never develops properly. To get from point A to point B, the child ends up pushing off from the side of the foot, like a skater, or rolling the weight to the outside edge.

Kids love to go barefooted and so do many adults. They don't realize it but they are listening to their bodies. The foot wants freedom. Encourage your children to go without their shoes when weather and other conditions permit. It will help them develop balance and agility.

DEVELOPMENTAL STAGES

We can learn a lot from children. But we've got to open our eyes and look at what they're doing (or not doing). The infant lying on its back, toes wiggling, fingers twiddling, arms flapping about is showing us the very first stage of functional development. This marvelous mechanism, which is the human body, is literally beginning at the beginning. The child is awakening his peripheral muscles, programming those muscles, from a horizontal supine position. Gravity is pressing down but otherwise there is no friction or interference from the environment.

As the baby's legs and arms start moving more and more, the major muscle groups come into play. Development shifts from the outside, the periphery of the body, to the inside. At this point, he flips over onto his stomach into a horizontal prone position like a swimmer. Now the body's geometry is put to use—the S-curve of the spine and the pelvic arch—in combination with the major muscles. The increase in tactile stimulation from being belly-down prompts more wiggling and jiggling. There is increased friction and resistance, which, as the child twists and turns and reaches out, provides a heavier workout for the muscles.

The next phase is called horizontal load-bearing. The baby pushes up onto his hands and knees. Bingo! The spine is activated. The hips and shoulders go to work. In very short order, horizontal load-bearing evolves into vertical load-bearing. The child stands on two feet.

The human infant is born with all the necessary bipedal functions. In the first weeks and months and years of life, those functions are discovered by random movement and then deliberately put to use in response to the mental and physical needs of the child within the context of his environment.

In terms of my outline of the child's developmental stages, what would happen if the environment encouraged or demanded that baby remain on its back in the horizontal supine position? Would it be standing on two feet?

No way. The child has to get over onto its stomach to continue developing the muscles and functions to move on to the next stage. Luckily the environment, and parents are part of the environment, tends not to get in the way. But things start going wrong in the horizontal prone position and the horizontal load-bearing position. If you strap the baby into a car seat, hold it for hours on end, bundle it up for long rides in the pram or in one of those contraptions that allows Dad or Mom to jog while pushing the kid along like a set of golf clubs, then what's happening? The environment starts restricting motion, development, and function.

Let me offer a vivid example of restricted motion. I now have a patient who is in his mid-thirties. As an infant he was diagnosed as suffering from cerebral palsy. And true enough, John had gone through a traumatic birth. Some oxygen deprivation slowed the development of his physical functions. But instead of going back and working to awaken those functions and get him physically up to speed, the boy (and the man) was treated as a cerebral palsy victim. Nobody expected him to function normally and therefore he didn't.

In two days of work at the clinic, John was able to get up and down stairs without assistance and without the characteristic lurching side-to-side walk that we associate with the cerebral palsy condition. John could have done that when he was eight years old. Instead he had to wait until he was nearly thirty-five.

THE CURSE OF THE FUZZY BUNNY

Infants are a handful and it's understandable when parents get nervous as a child goes into its crawling phase, "Look out! . . . What's the baby doing?" Man is a problem solver. A crawling infant is a problem. The solution is to either see to it that the child is in a space that is free of hazard, or to restrict the space in some way. That's why playpens were invented; then there's the old standby of surrounding little Jessica with toys and books and stuffed animals to keep her amused and in one place. What we've done to Jessica is to encourage her to restrict her own movement. She doesn't have to use her hands and knees and shoulders to scoot over to check out the mail slot in the front door, or investigate the dog's dish. She's got a fuzzy bunny right beside her to cuddle and dozens of other things to pick up and put down while sitting on her bottom.

Mom and Dad have created an environment that discourages movement.

SHOW AND TELL

Spin your homemade videotape ahead on fast forward to the pre-teen and teen years. In the interim there have been hundreds of hours of watching "Sesame Street" on television and countless Saturday mornings of cartoon shows. I can't believe that somehow our culture has convinced parents that "Sesame Street" is better for their children's development than being outside running and jumping and climbing and rolling around on the grass. But it's happened and we are paying the price.

Want to take a quick look at the bill? Ask your son or daughter to come out in the backyard and do a little monkey business on a tree limb or swing set. When they hang by their hands off the ground, you'll see the effects of "Sesame Street," playpens, fuzzy bunnies, years of sitting in a car or at a school desk. There will be many symptoms of dysfunction. One leg might be shorter than another. The right leg may dangle out in front of the left. A hip could be high. The feet could splay outward.

I don't mean to pick on "Sesame Street." Lack of motion in our environment and culture is the culprit. When I make that statement in front of a live audience, I'm usually asked, "Fine . . . how much motion should our children have in the course of a day? An hour, two hours?"

Thirty or forty years ago, probably when you were young, children were out running around all day long in the summer. Mothers had all they could do to get their kids to come in for dinner or bed. Psychologists and anthropologists say man functions at his best when he arises at dawn and goes to sleep at dusk. Only hunger and fatigue limit a healthy child's capacity—and craving— for physical activity.

Today many suburban neighborhoods seem like ghost towns on the weekends and after school. Where are the children? Well, they're taking special tutoring to pass the pre-SATs, attending music lessons, going out for PeeWee football practice, messing with the computer, flipping hamburgers at McDonald's for spending money, riding around in a friend's new car, watching TV, playing Nintendo.

I suggest you do an informal time and motion study on your child. If the "down time" to "go time" ratio exceeds 50 percent, it's advisable to look for ways to readjust the balance. While you're at it, conduct a similar study on yourself. "Do as I say not as I do" has never been a sound rule of effective parenting. Adults must modify their own lifestyles to include more, much more, movement. If youngsters grow up participating with their parents in physical activity, they'll tend to stay active, the reason being that they've been allowed to develop and maintain their design functions. Movement becomes a habit, a pleasurable habit that fuels the youngster's sense of self confidence and well-being.

OLD GLORY

To better understand what's happening to our children it's instructive to take a look at the elderly.

If I'm having a rough day in my clinic I'll look down at my list of appointments to see if a client over the age of fifty is scheduled to visit. The prospect always improves my spirits. It's like climbing into a time machine and visiting the past.

Older people are generally in better functional shape than their children and grandchildren. There are aches and pains and dysfunctions, but I have found that those who came of age in the 1950s and earlier recover faster from many injuries and are more readily able to systematically restore lost functions.

One reason for this is that as children, they were allowed to develop all the design functions of the body by running and jumping, twisting and turning. The environment of forty, fifty, sixty years ago encouraged motion. We've all probably heard Grandad's story about walking five miles to school through swirling blizzards. Or was it ten miles and pounding hailstones?

Exaggeration aside, there is a large element of truth to the tale. To get an education, to go to work, to make a living, or to have some fun, our grandparents were required to move.

I am forty-five, and my parents' generation, those in their seventies and eighties today, were the last to grow up without television, the modern ball and chain. The thirty to fifty hours a week that children now spend in front of the TV is thirty to fifty hours less time for physical activity. I can observe the signs of that activity in the knees and shoulders, hips and feet of the elderly.

STRENGTH TO STRENGTH

I'm sure you've heard this comment or variations on it: "Dad was fine until he retired but then went down hill real fast."

Given the observable functional superiority of the elderly, I believe there is a direct correlation linking retirement, the resulting lack of motion and subsequent geriatric illness. Reintroducing the elderly to motion is the quickest and cheapest way to fight cancer, heart disease, and diabetes.

For starters, researchers have found a link between exercise and the immune system—and what a place to start! The body's immune system is the first line of defense against cancer and other diseases; mysteriously enough, it can also end up being the first line of offense. When things go terribly wrong, the immune system literally destroys the body to save it.

Researchers have struggled for years to understand the reasons for the immune system's Jekyll and Hyde personality. There are many different theories. My explanation is that the immune system is motion-dependent, like all the other systems of the body. Therefore, it is weakened and disoriented by lack of motion. Physicians at the UCLA School of Medicine have found that the activity of a type of white blood cell, tagged NK cells for "natural killer" cells, is stimulated by moderate exercise. Without exercise, the NK cells are not up to the job of defending the body. Thus, carcinogens get a head start; the NK cells, sensing that they are at a disadvantage, pile on in overreaction.

A healthy immune system, one that is nourished by motion, can deliver its cancer fighting cells in a measured response, gradually escalating the countermeasures to match the threat. The "bug" is hit with a fly swatter, not a sledgehammer.

The same UCLA research team also discovered that the immune systems of elderly people in good health are sounder, and actually superior to the systems of individuals half their age.

The finding does not bode well for the young and the dysfunctional. It suggests to me that when the aging "baby boomers" enter their sixties and seventies, for those who last that long, the odds of surviving cancer will be more unfavorable for them than it was for their parents. By living at least part of their lives in an environment that required motion, older people had the chance to bring their bodily systems on-line and to strengthen them. Their children and grandchildren haven't been so lucky.

DRUG-FREE

There have been a number of studies demonstrating that exercise is also effective in controlling moderately elevated blood pressure. What's even more interesting is a recent test that turned up evidence that exercise is as effective as drugs in actually lowering blood pressure. Fifty-two men with mild hypertension were divided into three groups: The first group received a drug known as a beta-blocker, the second got a calcium channel blocker, and the third took a placebo. All of them participated in a ten-week exercise program that included aerobics and weight training.

The blood pressure of the placebo group dropped from an average of 145/97 to 131/84. Those taking the drugs had similar reductions, which prompted the researchers to say, "There was no added benefit to the use of either drug in these patients."

The study should have been front-page news all across the country. But the medical community didn't get very excited about it, and for good reason. Physicians know that it is easier for their hypertense patients to take drugs—and to take them every day for the rest of their lives—then it is to participate in a regular exercise routine. Many patients prefer the drugs to the exercise program.

It's easier. Easier to take drugs than to take a walk, take a run, take a turn around the dance floor? Easier than a half-hour with an exercise routine drawn from chapter five? If so, the time has come for a serious attitude reappraisal.

GAS AND GO

Between 1980 and 1987, the incidence of diabetes in the United States rose by 17 percent. Federal researchers at the Centers for Disease Control broke the figures down by sex and race. They found that the number of white men with diabetes mellitus increased by 33 percent during the time period. The CDC scientists think the increase is related to the aging of America. But I don't agree.

The incidence of diabetes among white females was unchanged. A 33 percent spread between men and women is hard to reconcile, given that both sexes are riding the crest of the same demographic wave. I believe what we're seeing is another example of a motion-sensitive bodily system being adversely affected by our sedentary and dysfunctional lifestyle.

The body has an ingenious and complex method for maintaining its "fuel" levels. Essentially, our engines run on glucose, which results from the way the digestive system converts the food we eat. No glucose, no energy (except when we are burning off our fat supply).

Therefore, the body keeps close tabs on input and output. When we overeat and underexercise, instead of generating an unnecessary supply of glucose, some of the excess is converted to glycogen, a starch, and stored away in the muscles and liver to be available on demand for the next day's hunting and gathering. But the remaining extra glucose must also be dealt with. One of the mechanisms for regulating the glucose supply in the bloodstream is the pancreas; it functions as the enforcer or hit man. After an extra handful of elk meat is converted into glucose that won't be used—the hunter rolls over and takes a nap—the pancreas then goes into action. It releases insulin to burn off or convert the glucose. Ten thousand years ago, the pancreatic hit man rarely needed to get tough because the supply and demand for glucose was in balance. But the pancreas was always there just in case of a glucose overload.

The body, being a marvelously efficient machine, does not do any more work than it has to, and digestion is a lot of work. When a cheap and abundant supply of fuel comes along in the form of pure sugar, it doesn't bother going to the trouble of converting, processing, and sorting. The sugar is passed directly into the bloodstream as instant glucose. Luckily, primitive man did not encounter megadoses of sugar all that often. Perhaps there was an occasional snack of honeycomb that a bear obligingly dug out of a beehive. When it happened, the pancreas got real pushy and sucked up sugar as fast as it could, even to the point of absorbing necessary glucose and throwing our ancestors into a honey hangover.

Anybody who has been in a room full of hyperactive five year olds on sugar highs can readily imagine the consequences of a tribe of hunter-gatherers wired up on bellies full of honey. Maybe that's where the term "sweet-tooth" comes from.

Now, we go from the cave to the family room. Dad has just finished a Pepsi and the peanut-brittle left over from Christmas while watching "Monday Night Football" on TV. The pancreas springs into action. Actually, I should say the pancreas limps into action. The glucose hit man has had a long day. It started early with a jelly doughnut and a cup of coffee brimming with cream and sugar. At mid-morning there was a second cup of coffee and half a danish pastry. Throughout the day, the pancreas was run ragged with "pick-me-ups" of coffee, Cokes, and candy. Meanwhile, the body's blood sugar level went through a series of spikes and troughs. Dad is on his way to joining that 33 percent increase in white male diabetes victims.

Mom, on the other hand, is not. Why? She watches her weight, participates in an aerobics dance class (women have been the fitness trendsetters in recent years from power-walking to weight lifting), and, in addition to a nine-to-five job, does the bulk of the child-rearing and household chores. Supermom.

Factoring out the weight-watching, Mom's diet is probably similar to Dad's. There is a cultural imperative that determines what we eat. Men and women are equally influenced by it, equally trapped in a sugar-coated world. But Mom is still moving and, as a result, her system for regulating blood sugar levels is more functional.

ARTHRITIS

An estimated 37 million Americans have arthritis. Although the disease strikes every age group, it is commonly thought of as a malady that occurs more frequently among the elderly.

One theory about arthritis is that it's caused by a malfunctioning immune system. Something happens to trigger a white blood cell response, powerful substances are secreted into the joints, there's inflammation, swelling, and, in the most severe cases, destruction and deformation of bone, ligament, and cartilage.

As I said earlier in this chapter, a healthy immune system depends on motion. The causal chain that leads to arthritis may, indeed, begin with an environment that restricts movement. Once it gains a foothold, the disease perpetuates itself by crippling the victim. The joint that doesn't move in a functional way and in sufficient amounts becomes one that cannot move at all, further goading the immune system into a disproportionate response.

Arthritis seems to seek out the quietest places in the body. What could be better than a cozy joint capsule that doesn't get all that much use in the course of a day? Obligingly, the synovial membrane that surrounds the joint begins to flood the capsule with fluid at the first sign of the white cell invasion. The synovia's job, after all, is to lubricate the joint and, failing that, to inject so much lubricant that it is water-logged to a point of complete immobility. Hence, the arthritis settles back comfortably in its own version of a hot tub.

Medical researchers have found that white blood cells will assault heart muscle tissue that is deprived of oxygen during a heart attack. The same thing may be happening in joints with arthritis. An inactive joint is not properly oxygenated. The body will not waste metabolic resources on a joint, an organ, a muscle, or connective tissue that it senses is not performing. Each part of the body only gets exactly what's called for to accomplish the task it's required to do. In this way, the body is both a classic capitalist and an orthodox marxist when the time comes to distribute the wealth: Each according to his need and no work, no pay.

The white blood cells are going after the joint in the same way they pounce on deoxygenated heart muscle tissue. Even though the doctors have revived the heart attack victim, the white cells consider the tissue to be dead and, therefore, of great danger to the living if it is not disposed of immediately. By the same token, the joints are written off as dead zones to be cleaned out with heavy doses of caustic substances.

Maintaining adequate movement, therefore, is essential. With arthritis there seems to be gradual escalation of the white cell attack that may correlate with the pace of the ensuing immobilization. Thus, the less the victim moves, the worse the arthritis becomes. As motion decreases because of the arthritis pain, the white cells get meaner and meaner until they go into a final feeding frenzy.

HARD SELL

Arthritis hurts, and unlike other musculoskeletal disorders the pain is not as easily suppressed by the reintroduction of proper design-function movement. I can readily convince a new client to spend a half hour a day doing exercises if he or she has just been relieved of excruciating back spasm pain after a couple of minutes spent lying on the floor doing a static back press. But I work hard to prepare an arthritis sufferer psychologically to realize that progress measured in inches, as opposed to miles, is still progress.

Giving in to the temptation to rely on drugs and joint replacement surgery is understandable as a means of gaining relief from pain. However, without reintroducing motion to the arthritis victim, the immune system remains in a weakened condition and the rest of the body's joints are still sitting there waiting for the disease to come along and post the do-not-disturb signs.

To compound the problem, many of the drugs that are prescribed for arthritis, aspirin being an old standby, restrict the bloodstream's ability to carry oxygen. By thinning out the blood, the joints get even less oxygen than they did before the treatment began. Thus, there's a real danger that a vicious cycle will whirl out of control and trigger more arthritis, the need for more drugs, another round of surgical intervention, and on and on.

PRIME OR PAIN

Between the young and the elderly, there is a vast territory that is harder to label. It should be called "Prime Time," but for many us it is pain time.

Like the athlete who blames his pain on the sport he is playing, there is a tendency to attribute sore backs and wrists, aching necks and knees to conditions in the workplace or at home.

Mattresses are the all-time favorite culprit, and I am also constantly being told by patients that the desk chair at the office is causing their bad backs. "Why is it," I ask in reply, "that clerks in Victorian-era law offices and counting houses sat on high flat stools that didn't even have backs on them? And they did it ten hours a day." A huge industry has grown up in recent years to make and sell ergonomically correct office furniture. The assumption is that something is wrong—ergonomically incorrect—with the desks and the chairs that we've been using.

There is nothing wrong with the furniture. What's wrong is that our bodies are dysfunctional.

The back is designed to support itself. The chair and its support, or lack thereof, are irrelevant. The back is designed to bear its own weight without help from foam rubber or tufted leather.

BOTTOMLESS

When we stand or sit, the muscles of the body are still moving. Just standing upright and maintaining our balance requires the effort of about three hundred muscles. When we plop down into a fancy desk chair, our lower torsos say, "Terrific . . . let's take a break." The chair becomes a surrogate for the feet, the legs, the gluteal muscles, and the flexor muscles of the lower back. The intricately varied gradations of alternating contraction and relaxation subside. From the waist down, the other systems of the body are left to function on their own; circulation, digestion, and elimination all suffer.

The upper torso, meantime, doesn't know anything about the chair. It continues to contract and relax as if the lower torso was fully engaged. The pelvis, caught in the middle, starts to compensate. Our superbly flexible shoulders are no match for the powerful hip flexor-extensor-adductor muscles. It is only a matter of time before we lose our parallel lines—head over the shoulders, shoulders over the hips, hips over the knees, and knees over the ankles.

The fancy chair does to our torso what expensive running shoes do to the feet. Just as the sole of the shoe is a platform that prevents the foot from coming into direct contact with the ground, where it can analyse the contours of the terrain and adjust the appropriate muscles from head to toe, the chair forces the upper torso to perform an unnatural act: balance itself on the end of the spine, a job that it was not designed to do.

The stiffness and soreness that we feel after sitting down are the muscles sending us a message: "The body is a unit. Get the lower torso off its butt!"

What do we do? We get a new chair, one that will cradle the lower back and stop it from hurting. Eventually, we trade up to a more impressive "throne" that allows the suffering spinal column and shoulders to lean over like the tower of Pisa while we tap away at the keyboard, read, or make phone calls.

The chair is taking on more and more functions. To stop the Tower of Pisa from toppling over and falling out of the chair entirely, some muscles go into permanent contraction. It's like the last man on the rope belaying a party of mountain climbers moving across a dangerous slope. But in this case, the climbers are all plunging down the mountain. As it struggles to stop the free-fall, the muscle screams in pain.

REPETITIVE MOTION

Shoulder dysfunction, not carpal tunnel syndrome or a grab bag of other hand, wrist, forearm, and elbow disorders that are lumped together as repetitive strain injury (RSI), is the cause of what's being described as the new epidemic of the workplace. In 1989, the U.S. Labor Department reported that repetitive motion injuries increased by almost 30 percent compared to 1988 and accounted for more than half of all occupational illness. Former Labor Secretary Elizabeth Hanford Dole described repetitive motion injuries as "one of the nation's greatest worker health and safety concerns in the decade of the 1990s." Mrs. Dole's department persuaded General Motors and the United Auto Workers to cooperate in an effort to eliminate what the head of the Occupational Safety and Health Administration said were the root causes of repetitive motion trauma. In announcing the program, the official said that tools and assembly line work stations would be redesigned and mechanical devices developed to prevent excessive heavy lifting.

Root causes? Tools, work stations, excessive heavy lifting? It's a variation on blaming the desk chair or the soft mattress or the cramped airline seat. Apply the information about function and dysfunction that you've gathered so far from this book and look around your own workplace with an eye to predicting who among your colleagues will end up with carpal tunnel syndrome or other repetitive-motion disorders.

Is there one characteristic that stands out?

Slumping shoulders.

Shoulders rolled forward and locked in the hinged position are an invitation to repetitive-motion trauma. The tendons in the arm must have free passage. Like a kink in a garden hose that cuts off the flow of water, the dysfunctional shoulder is restricting and irritating the tendons.

New tools and more comfortable work stations may delay the onset of carpal tunnel syndrome and RSI by suppressing the symptomatic pain, but what's happening is that the remedy essentially consists of a further reduction in motion—the tool or work station is doing more of the moving—without addressing the correctable dysfunction. As always, the "cure," when it involves less movement, is worse than the disease. Less motion is not more happiness and health. Less is less. Unless the dysfunction is addressed, the worker with RSI is caught in a downward spiral. Each new tool and work station begets another new tool and work station to accommodate the accumulating dysfunctions that result from lack of motion. Finally, the day arrives when we hear, "Too bad. The American worker just can't hack it anymore. . . . We'll just have to go to Europe or Asia or Latin American to find employees who can do the work." In New England this used to be called "going south," when the textile mills migrated to the Carolinas and Georgia chasing cheap labor and low taxes. But going south isn't going to work much longer as Mexico, the rest of Central and Latin America, Asia and Europe also succumb to the good life—the good and motionless life.

THE MOVING FINGER

To understand carpal tunnel syndrome and other RSI disorders, try this exercise. Put your hand and forearm flat, palm down, on the desk in front of you. Move away from the desk a little with your back erect. Get comfortable.

You should notice an arch under your wrist. The heel of the hand, forearm and elbow come in contact with the desk, but not the underside of the wrist.

Slide in closer to the desk while keeping your wrist where it is. Hunch the shoulders and roll them forward. What happens? First, your shoulder blade lets you know that it's part of the unit. There was probably a tightening near the rotator cuff area. Most importantly, though, you should have noticed that the arch in the wrist flattened out as the heel of the hand was pressed downward and the forearm hinged upward.

By asking you to move from a functional to an overtly dysfunctional position, I have provoked the bones, muscles, and tendons in your wrist, shoulder, and arm to compensate. They are violating the design of the body.

Wiggle your fingers. The muscles and the connective tissue, the ligaments, the tendons, and the articulation of the hands and the fingers are all designed for a downstroke with the fine muscles of the hand doing the work, not the tendons and muscles of the forearm.

Look at the face of your wristwatch. Keep looking at it. The hand will start to drop lower than the wrist and forearm. And that's the position it is supposed to be in, knuckles lower than the wrist, otherwise the muscles of the forearm take over. If you put your arm back on the table, palm down, the only way to flatten the wrist is to push downward at the shoulder. Thus, hunching over with the shoulder forward automatically flattens the arch at the wrist. The forearm muscles are now jerking up and down like a bell rope struggling to make the fingers work, and they don't like all that effort. A protest is registered at the head office in the form of inflammation and pain.

Sit at the keyboard and type. First with your shoulders back, then hunched over. You are actually pushing the wrist down and away. Some people compound the problem by cocking their wrist and hands into that position, thinking that will counteract the fatigue and lack of control that sets in after typing a while. In reality, it's making everything worse.

The typical remedy is to put a brace on the wrist or rig up a contraption on the keyboard to hold the wrist in the proper—that is, painless—position. If that doesn't work the choices come down to unemployment disability or surgery.

Susan rejected both options. She is a teacher who works with the deaf using sign language. When her hands started going numb, the state of California decided that they would either pay for an operation or put Susan on permanent disability due to carpal tunnel syndrome. She insisted on coming in to see me first. The disability officials fought the idea, but Susan kicked up a fuss and they gave in. Three months later, after weekly two-hour visits to the clinic, she was back at work. And her shoulders were back in position.

No drugs, no surgery—no disability payments.

9

Volume Control

I almost didn't write this book because I was concerned that something would get lost on the printed page. And maybe it has. There is no substitute for the Socratic method, practiced one-on-one.

In my clinic, first I explain the body's design, and then I ask questions: "Where's your weight? On your heels or on the balls of your feet? If you suffer from TMJ pain, why doesn't it hurt right now? How come your congested sinuses opened up after you did that exercise?" Those questions force people to interact with their own experience. In a flash they understand how critical motion and function are to the body.

I can't do that in a book unless the reader catches on quickly and realizes that it isn't enough to just follow the logic of my argument. You've got to immediately experience the effect. The shock of recognition is essential. It goes well beyond intellectual perception and goes right to the emotions and instincts. You must *feel* your own body responding.

The only reason I included the material in chapters four and five was to give you the opportunity to step through the mirror in your own bedroom and walk into my clinic. I did not want this book to be another workout or fitness manual. Nor did I want it to be a "pain book." There are already enough of those and they haven't solved the problem. The exercises are here along with the illustrations just in case the words—tens of thousands more than I ever need in the clinic—managed to tap your powers of intuition, judgment, motivation, and experience. If so, you've started to feel

and "hear" your body again; the exercises will turn up the volume
until the messages are coming through loud and clear.

A VARSITY LETTER

In the spring of 1989, I got a telephone call from a young man by
the name of Mark Adickes. At the time he was a lineman for the
Kansas City Chiefs (he's now with the Washington Redskins).
Mark's back was hurting him badly and he wanted to know if he
could drive down from Los Angeles to see me. It was Sunday and
I was at home, but there was no way I could say, "How about
tomorrow?" I could feel the pain coming down the phone line.

When Mark arrived, I put him down on my living room floor in
the static back position. It took two hours, but finally the pain
subsided.

Mark Adickes wrote me a letter in 1990 which demonstrates
what I am talking about when I say that the Egoscue Method
"turns up the volume."

Midway through the 1987 season I began to develop back pain.
My back pain was diagnosed by the team doctor as "linesman's
back," caused by weak back muscles and normal wear and tear. He
prescribed a series of oral cortisone pills and recommended a vigorous off-season weight lifting program to strengthen the back. In
the summer of 1988, upon completion of my weight training my
back was worse, only now it was accompanied by leg pain. In this
condition I began the running phase of my conditioning. During
the first workout . . . I injured my back more severely. I was just
finishing a 440 when I felt as if I had been stabbed in the lower
back with a knife.

At this point I was in a state of panic. Training camp was less
than a month away and I could barely walk. During this month I
saw five chiropractors, two acupuncturists, three masseuses, four
different physical therapists, an acupressurist, and a Feldenkrais
worker [this is a therapeutic technique based on the belief that an
individual can be trained to consciously control his or her own
central nervous system to enhance motor skills and thereby counteract dysfunctions of the musculoskeletal system]. All these caused
little or no improvement. I began training camp to prepare for the
1988 season knowing my whole career was in jeopardy. On the

first day of camp, in the first contact drill, I reinjured my back hitting a dummy.

After a thorough doctor's examination, including a CAT scan, it was concluded I had Spondylolisthesis with a bulging disk. The team physician recommended a series of cortisone shots. I opted for a second opinion and traveled to Los Angeles to see the back specialists at Doctor Jobe's Centinella Hospital clinic. After further testing, including MRI, CTI, and a Mylogram, the same remedy was prescribed with spinal fusion as the alternative. I traveled back to Kansas City and was given a series of four cortisone epidural blocks over a two-week period and a rehabilitation workout consisting of spine neural trunk stabilizing exercises.

I missed the rest of the 1988 preseason as well as the first six games of the regular season before I returned rehabilitated. I was stiff and immobile with a significant loss of balance. The pain quickly returned and I struggled through the remainder of the season taking pain killers and anti-inflammatories like they were "Flintstone's chewables." At my post-season physical I was told that spinal fusion was inevitable if I didn't improve. At this point I was contemplating retirement rather than risk back surgery at the ripe old age of twenty-seven.

Upon my calling my college strength coach to relay the news of my impending retirement, I learned of the Egoscue Method. The Chiefs sent me to Los Angeles to work with Centinella's physical therapists. Prior to leaving Kansas City, I called Pete Egoscue to set up an appointment. After two days of therapy [at Centinella's] without improvement, I drove down to San Diego from L.A. I could barely walk when I emerged from the car. Just by watching the way I stood and walked, Pete diagnosed my problem as severe hip dysfunction, and put me on a program to correct it. After my first two hours, using the Egoscue Method, I was pain-free for the first time in over two years. The program I was given called for routines in the morning and evening and with each successive workout the pain stayed away longer and I could see the functions return to my body. The Egoscue Method identified and isolated the root of my problem. It not only relieved my pain but made me feel younger and more vital as the body returned to anatomical alignment.

I have just completed the 1989 season injury-free and with an ever brighter future. If I continue to improve at my present rate I could play until I'm forty years old. The knee pain I used to experience daily is gone along with the back pain. Long-distance running, which used to be impossible, is now a joy. At 280 pounds I can also run more than six miles without developing sore ankles and knees. The Egoscue Method has given me a new lease on life in a rough neighborhood called the NFL.

MARK ADICKES

Turning up the volume? "It not only relieved my pain but made me feel younger and more vital as the body returned to anatomical alignment." A little guidance and *permission* was all Mark Adickes needed. I say permission because he already knew what was wrong and what had to be done to set it right, but he needed somebody to come along and back him up: "You don't need the spinal fusion, what you need is to get your body back into the shape it was when you were nineteen and it didn't hurt."

MAX, MOM, AND MOTION

Last fall I got a letter from a mother whose son was born with his umbilical cord wrapped around his neck. The doctors managed to save the infant but there was acute oxygen deprivation. She told me the boy was eleven years old and in a wheelchair. Cerebral palsy was the diagnosis, since his mental and physical development had been severely retarded.

Her letter explained that Max had worked with the best doctors and therapists and that he was a real fighter. Over the years he had made slow and steady progress, but still had a long, long way to go. She said her son had set a goal that he would walk by the time he was thirteen. At eleven, they were beginning to run out of time.

Max's mother had heard that I helped injured athletes and other individuals restore lost function. She said Max had all of his normal functions prior to the accident that occurred at birth. Would I see him?

Max came into the clinic with his mom in early December of 1990. She was right—he's a fighter. But he was a little boy with big problems.

We put him on the floor and literally turned back the clock to infancy. I wanted him to try crawling back and forth. It was tough. The next day his mother reported that Max's abdominal muscles were really hurting.

It was like hearing that I had just won a twenty million dollar lottery jackpot. The pain was telling me that a dormant function had been reawakened. The boy had his functions, they just weren't being used. As a diagnosed victim of cerebral palsy, he was treated like one from the day he was born. He was held and carried and put in a wheelchair. Max got bigger; his legs and arms grew, but the muscles and kinesthetic sense lagged way behind, having never been engaged in the first place, or having been used only minimally.

After a few more days in the clinic, I sent Max home with a menu of exercises, and I went cross-country skiing over the holiday period. One afternoon, the office called to tell me the news: Max walked for the first time on Christmas day 1990.

Now you know why I like my job. Now you know why I wrote this book.

Notes and Sources

CHAPTER ONE

For general myology data: Fritz Kahn, M.D., *Man in Structure and Function*, Vol. I, translated and edited by George Rosen, M.D. New York: Alfred A. Knopf, 1947.

CHAPTER THREE

The definition of cartilage is in part drawn from *Steadman's Medical Dictionary*, 25th Edition, Williams & Wilkins, 1990.

The properties of cartilage, including the findings that the tissue is altered by exercise, is covered in Jurgen Weinecks' *Functional Anatomy in Sports*, Mosby Year Book, 1990.

CHAPTER SEVEN

The possibility of neurological damage from high-impact aerobics is reported in "Doctor Says High-Impact Aerobics Can Cause Vertigo," Associated Press, *Washington Post*, December 8, 1990.

CHAPTER EIGHT

Norman Cousins' *Head First: The Biology of Hope* (New York: Penguin, 1989) discusses the immune system and research findings regarding an increase in NK cell activity after moderate exercise; see page 238. Also, in the same discussion, Cousins deals with the immune system in older patients as compared to the young.

Blood pressure and exercise are dealt with in an article titled "Is Exercise the Cure for High Blood Pressure?" in the *Wellness Letter* (University of California, Berkeley, August 1990), Vol. 6, issue 11, p. 1.

Federal research on diabetes rates is reported in the *Washington Post*, December 4, 1990 (AP dispatch).

The data on the number of arthritis sufferers are taken from the Arthritis Foundation, *Understanding Arthritis*, Irving Kishner, M.D., editor (New York: Scribner's, 1984). Also, material on the disease process was drawn from this source.

White blood cell attacks on heart muscle tissue and joints is drawn from *The New York Times*, "Molecules that Direct Immune System Traffic Excite Researchers," December 4, 1990, p. C3.

CHAPTER NINE

Letter, January 1990, from Mark Adickes to Pete Egoscue.

Index